# Biostatistics and Epidemiology

Sylvia Wassertheil-Smoller

# Biostatistics and Epidemiology

## A Primer for Health Professionals

With 20 illustrations

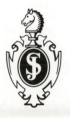

Springer-Verlag
New York  Berlin  Heidelberg
London  Paris  Tokyo  Hong Kong

SYLVIA WASSERTHEIL-SMOLLER
Albert Einstein College of Medicine
1300 Morris Park Avenue, Room 1312
Bronx, NY 10461, USA

Library of Congress Cataloging-in-Publication Data
Wassertheil-Smoller, Sylvia.
    Biostatistics & epidemiology : a primer for health professionals /
Sylvia Wassertheil-Smoller.
        p.      cm.
    Includes bibliographical references.
    Includes index.
    ISBN 0-387-97312-5 (alk. paper)
    1. Epidemiology — Statistical methods.   2. Clinical trials-
-Statistical methods.   I. Title.   II. Title: Biostatistics and
epidemiology.
    [DNLM:   1. Biometry.   2. Epidemiologic Methods.     WA 950 W322b]
RA652.2.M3W37      1990
614.4′072 — dc20
DNLM/DLC
for Library of Congress                                         90-9748
                                                                  CIP

Printed on acid-free paper

Camera-ready copy provided by the author.
Printed and bound by Edwards Brothers, Inc., Ann Arbor, MI.
Printed in the United States of America.

9  8  7  6  5  4  3  2  1

ISBN 0-387-97312-5 Springer-Verlag New York Berlin Heidelberg
ISBN 3-540-97312-5 Springer-Verlag Berlin Heidelberg New York

*To Jordan*

# PREFACE

This book is intended to be non-threatening to those who have limited or no background in mathematics and thus there are a minimum of formulae. The presentation of the material is aimed to give an understanding of the underlying principles, as well as practical guidelines of "how to do it" and "how to interpret it." The topics included are those which are most commonly used or referred to, in the literature.

I hope this book will be useful to diverse groups of people in the health field, as well as to those in related areas. The material is intended for 1) physicians doing clinical research as well as for those doing basic research; 2) for students - medical, college and graduate; 3) for research staff in various capacities; and 4) for anyone interested in the logic and methodology of biostatistics and epidemiology. The principles and methods described here are applicable to various substantive areas, including medicine, public health, psychology and education. Of course, not all topics which are specifically relevant to each of these disciplines, can be covered in this short text.

There are some features to note which may aid the reader in the use of this book:

a) The book starts with a discussion of the philosophy and logic of science and the underlying principles of testing what we believe against the reality of our experiences. While such a discussion, per se, will not help the reader to actually "do a t-test", I think it is important to provide some introduction to the underlying framework of the field of epidemiology and statistics, to understand why we do what we do.

b) Many of the subsections stand alone, i.e. the reader can turn to the topic that interests him or her and read the material out of sequential order. This is done so that the book may be used by those who need it for special purposes. The reader is free to skip those topics which are not of interest without being too much hampered in further reading. As a result there is some redundancy. In my teaching experience, however, I have found that it is better to err on the side of redundancy than on the side of sparsity.

c) Cross-references to other relevant sections are included when additional explanation is needed.

d) When development of a topic is beyond the scope of this text, the reader is referred to other books which deal with the material in more depth or on a higher mathematical level. A list of recommended texts is provided in the back.

# ACKNOWLEDGEMENTS

I want to express my thanks to Dr. Jacob Cohen, whose inspired teaching started me on this path, to Jean Almond, who made it personally possible for me to continue on it, and to my colleagues and students at the Albert Einstein College of Medicine, who make it fun.

My appreciation goes to Dr. Brenda Breuer for her clear thinking and helpful suggestions, and to Dr. Ruth Hyman for giving of her time to review the statistics section and for making useful recommendations. I am very thankful to Dr. Ruth Macklin for her critique of the material on the logic of the scientific method and her scholarly urging for precision in thought and language.

I am greatly indebted to Rosemarie Sasso who has accomplished a remarkable feat in preparing this manuscript through multiple revisions, using her intelligence, skill and artistic sense, and always displaying good humor and unfailing patience.

Finally, my deep love and gratitude go to my husband Walter Austerer for his help and encouragement.

# CONTENTS

# *Section 3* - MOSTLY ABOUT STATISTICS

# *Section 5* - MOSTLY ABOUT CLINICAL TRIALS

*Section 1*

# THE SCIENTIFIC METHOD

*"Science is built up with facts, as a house is with stones.  But a collection of facts is no more a science than a heap of stones is a house."*
Jules Henri Poincare
La Science et l'Hypothese (1908)


## 1.1  The Logic of Scientific Reasoning

The whole point of science is to uncover the "truth".  How do we go about deciding something is true?  We have two tools as our disposal to pursue scientific inquiry:

We have our senses - through which we experience the world and make observations.

We have the ability to reason - which enables us to make logical inferences.

In science we impose logic on those observations.

Clearly, we need both tools.  All the logic in the world is not going to create an observation, and all the individual observations in the world, won't in themselves, create a theory.  There are two kinds of relationships between the scientific mind and the world - two kinds of logic we impose - *deductive and inductive*, as illustrated in Figure 1.1 below.

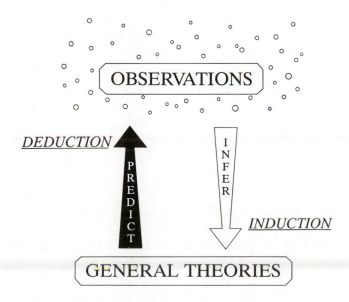

1

In *deductive inference*, we hold a theory and based on it we make a prediction of its consequences - i.e. we predict what the observations should be. For example, we may hold a theory of learning that says that positive reinforcement results in better learning than punishment - i.e. rewards work better than punishments. From this theory we predict that math students who are praised for their right answers during the year will do better on the final exam than those who are punished for their wrong answers. We go from the general - the theory - to the specific - the observations. This is known as the hypothetico-deductive method.

In *inductive inference,* we go from the specific to the general. We make many observations, discern a pattern, make a generalization, and infer an explanation. For example, it was observed in the Vienna General Hospital in the 1840's that women giving birth were dying at a high rate of puerperal fever, a generalization that provoked terror in prospective mothers. It was a young doctor called Ignaz Phillip Semmelweis who connected the observation that medical students performing vaginal examinations, did so directly after coming from the dissecting room, (rarely washing their hands in between), with the observation that a colleague who accidentally cut his finger while dissecting a corpse, died of a malady exactly like the one killing the mothers. He inferred the explanation that the cause of death was the introduction of cadaverous material into a wound. (The practical consequence of that creative leap of the imagination was the elimination of puerperal fever as a scourge of childbirth by requiring that physicians wash their hands before doing a delivery!) The ability to make such creative leaps from generalizations is the product of creative scientific minds.

Epidemiologists have generally been thought to use inductive inference. The following story is perhaps an apocryphal example of the creative leap of inductive inference. The receptionist in a doctor's office in California noted that the chairs on one side of the waiting room were all worn out at the edges of the seats. She told her bosses that she needed to recover them. This simple observation led the two doctors - one of whom happened to be a cardiologist - to wonder why just the edges of the seats on the right side of the room were worn. That was the side which was used by the cardiologist's patients. "You must have very strange patients," one of the doctors said to his cardiologist partner. And then they said -"EUREKA! All the patients who sit on this side of the room have heart disease. These people must have the kind of personality that makes them sit on the edge of their chairs, and they wear out the fabric. They must be very impatient and always in a hurry." And so the theory of the Type A personality leaped out at them. (It may not quite have happened that way, but it illustrates a point.) This theory, says in essence that men who are aggressively ambitious, driven, hostile, impatient, with a sense of time urgency and other associated personality characteristics, are more prone to heart attacks than those with a different personality.

However, there is another point to the story. Theories don't just leap out of facts. There must be some substrate out of which the theory leaps. Perhaps that substrate is another, preceding theory, which was found to be inadequate to explain these new observations, and that theory, in turn, had replaced some previous theory. In any case, one aspect of the "substrate" is the "prepared mind" of the cardiologist. He is trained to look at medical phenomena from a cardiology perspective and he is knowledgeable about preceding theories and their strengths and flaws. If he hadn't such training, he might not see the connection. Or if he had different training, he might leap to a different inference altogether. If he were trained as an infectious disease specialist, for example, he might come up with the theory that the patients harbor a virus on the seat of their pants that eats away the fabric of the chairs.

The question is how well does the theory hold up in the face of new observations? The Type A theory has a great deal of supportive evidence, though not all studies have corroborated the theory. Whether this is due to imperfect design and methodology of such studies or whether it is because the theory does not hold up, has not been established. Nevertheless, there have been many studies which have provided affirmative evidence in favor of the theory. Affirmative evidence means more examples which are consistent with the theory. But to what degree does supportive evidence strengthen an assertion? Those who believe induction is the appropriate logic of science, hold the view that affirmative evidence is what strengthens a theory.

Another approach is that of Karl Popper, perhaps one of the foremost theoreticians of science. Popper claims that induction arising from accumulation of affirmative evidence doesn't strengthen a theory. Induction after all is based on our belief that the things unobserved will be like those observed or that the future will be like the past. For example, we see a lot of white swans and we make the assertion that all swans are white. This assertion is supported by many observations. Each time we see another white swan, we have more supportive evidence. But we cannot prove that all swans are white no matter how many white swans we see. On the other hand, this assertion can be knocked down by the sighting of a single black swan. Now we would have to change our assertion to say that most swans are white and that there are some black swans. This assertion presumably is closer to the truth. In other words, we can refute the assertion with one example, but we can't prove it with many. (The assertion that all swans are white is a descriptive generalization rather than a theory. A theory has a richer meaning which incorporates causal explanations and underlying mechanisms. Assertions, like those relating to the color of swans, may be components of a theory).

According to Popper, the proper methodology is to posit a theory - or a conjecture, as he calls it, and try to demonstrate that it is false. The more such attempts at destruction it survives, the stronger is the evidence for it. The object is to devise ever more aggressive attempts to knock down the assertion and see if it still survives. If it does not survive an attempt at *falsification*, then the theory is discarded and replaced by another. He calls this the method of *conjectures and refutations*. The advance of science toward the "truth" comes about by discarding theories whose predictions are not confirmed by observations, or theories which are not testable altogether, (rather than by shoring up theories with more examples of where they work). *Useful scientific theories are potentially falsifiable.* Untestable theories are those where a variety of contradictory observations could each be consistent with the theory. For example, consider Freud's psychoanalytic theory. The Oedipal complex theory says that a child is in love with the parent of the opposite sex. A boy desires his mother and wants to destroy his father. If we observe a man to say he loves his mother, that fits in with the theory. If we observe a man to say he hates his mother, that also fits in with the theory which would say that it is "reaction formation" which leads him to deny his true feelings. In other words, no matter what the man says, it could not falsify the theory because it could be explained by it. Since no observation could potentially falsify the Oedipal theory, its position as a scientific theory could be questioned.

A third, and most reasonable view is that the progress of science requires both inductive and deductive inference. A particular point of view provides a framework for observations which lead to a theory which predicts new observations which modify the theory which then leads to new predicted observations and so on - towards the elusive "truth" - which we generally never reach. Asking which comes first, theory or observation, is like asking which comes first: the chicken or the egg.

In general then, advances in knowledge in the health field come about through constructing, testing and modifying theories. Epidemiologists make inductive inferences to generalize from many observations, make creative leaps of the imagination to infer explanations and construct theories, and use deductive inferences to test those theories.

Theories, then can be used to predict observations. But these observations will not always be exactly as we predict them, due to error and the inherent variability of natural phenomena. If the observations are widely different from our predictions we will have to abandon or modify the theory. How do we test the extent of the discordance of our predictions based on theory from the reality of our observations? The test is a statistical or probabilistic test. It is the test of *the null hypothesis which is the cornerstone of statistical inference* and which will be discussed later. Some excellent articles on the logic and philosophy of science, and applications in epidemiology, are listed in the bibliography at the end of this book.[1-5]

## 1.2 Variability of Phenomena Requires Statistical Analysis

Statistics is a methodology with broad areas of application in science and industry, as well as in medicine and in many other fields. A phenomenon may be principally based on a deterministic model. One example is Boyle's law, which states that for a fixed volume an increase in temperature of a gas determines that there is an increase in pressure. Each time this law is tested the same result occurs. The only variability lies in the error of measurement. Many phenomena in physics and chemistry are of such a nature.

Another type of model is a probabilistic model, which implies that various states of a phenomenon occur with certain probabilities. For instance, the distribution of intelligence is principally probabilistic, i.e., given values of intelligence occur with a certain probability in the general population. In biology, psychology, or medicine, where phenomena are influenced by many factors which in themselves are variable and by other factors which are unidentifiable, the models are often probabilistic. In fact, as knowledge in physics has become more refined, it begins to appear that models formerly thought to be deterministic are probabilistic.

In any case, where the model is principally probabilistic, statistical techniques are needed to increase scientific knowledge. *The presence of variation requires the use of statistical analysis.*[6] When there is little variation with respect to a phenomenon, much more weight is given to a small amount of evidence than where there is a great deal of variation. For example, we know that AIDS appears to be invariably a fatal disease. Thus, if we found a drug that indisputably cured a few patients of AIDS, we would give a lot of weight to the evidence that the drug represented a cure, far more weight than if the course of this disease were variable. In contrast to this example, if we were trying to determine whether Vitamin C cures colds, we would need to demonstrate its effect in many patients and we would need to use statistical methods to do so, since human beings are quite variable with respect to colds. In fact, in most biological and even more so in social and psychological phenomena, there is a great deal of variability.

## 1.3 Inductive Inference - Statistics as the Technology of the Scientific Method

Statistical methods are objective methods by which *group trends are abstracted from observations on many separate individuals.* A simple concept of statistics is the calculation of averages, percentages and so on and the presentation of data in tables and charts. Such techniques for summarizing data are very important indeed and essential to describing the population under study. However, they comprise a small part of the field of statistics. A major part of statistics involves the *drawing of inferences from samples to a population* in regard to some characteristic of interest. Suppose we are interested in the average blood pressure of women college students. If we could measure the blood pressure of every single member of this population, we would not have to infer anything. We would simply average all the numbers we obtained. In practice, however, we take a sample of students (properly selected) and on the basis of the data we obtain from the sample, we infer what the mean of the whole population is likely to be.

The reliability of such inferences or conclusions may be evaluated in terms of probability statements. In statistical reasoning then, we make inductive inferences - from the particular (sample) to the general (population). Thus, statistics may be said to be the technology of the scientific method.

## 1.4   Design of Studies

While the generation of hypotheses may come from anecdotal observations, the testing of those hypotheses must be done by making controlled observations, free of systematic bias. Statistical techniques, to be valid, must be applied to data obtained from well designed studies. Otherwise, solid knowledge is not advanced.

There are two types of studies: 1) Observational studies where "Nature" determines who is exposed to the factor of interest, and who is not exposed. These studies demonstrate association. Association may imply causation or it may not. 2) Experimental studies where the investigator determines who is exposed. These may prove causation.

Observational studies may be of three different study designs: *cross sectional, case-control, or prospective*. In a *cross-sectional study* the measurements are taken at one point in time. For example, in a cross sectional study of high blood pressure and coronary heart disease the investigators determine the blood pressure and the presence of heart disease at the same time and if they found an association, would not be able to tell which came first. Does heart disease result in high blood pressure or does high blood pressure cause heart disease, or are both high blood pressure and heart disease the result of some other common cause?

In a *case-control study* of smoking and lung cancer, for example, the investigator starts with cases of the disease, e.g., lung cancer, and with controls, and through examination of the records or through interviews, determines the presence or the absence of the factor in which he or she is interested (smoking). A case-control study is sometimes referred to as a *retrospective study* because data on the factor of interest is collected retrospectively, (and thus may be subject to various inaccuracies.)

In a *prospective (or cohort)* study the investigator starts with a cohort of non-diseased persons with that factor, (i.e., those who smoke) and persons without that factor, (nonsmokers), and goes forward into some future time to determine the frequency of development of the disease in the two groups. A prospective study is also known as a longitudinal study. *The distinction between case-control studies and prospective studies lies in the sampling. In the case-control study we sample from among the diseased and non-diseased while in a prospective study we sample from among those with the factor and those without the factor.* Prospective studies provide stronger evidence of causality than retrospective studies but are often more difficult, more costly and sometimes impossible to conduct, for example if the disease under study takes decades to develop, or if it is very rare.

In the health field, an experimental study to test an intervention of some sort is called a *clinical trial*. In a clinical trial the investigator assigns patients or participants to one group or another, usually randomly, while trying to keep all other factors constant, or controlled for, and compares the outcome of interest in the two (or more) groups. More about clinical trials is in Section 5.

In summary, then, the following are in ascending order of strength in terms of demonstrating causality:

*cross-sectional studies:* useful in showing associations, in providing early clues to etiology.

*case-control studies:* useful for rare diseases or conditions, or when the disease takes a very long time to become manifest (synonymous names: *retrospective studies*.)

*cohort studies:* useful for providing stronger evidence of causality, and less subject to biases due to errors of recall or measurement (synonymous names: *prospective studies, longitudinal studies*.)

*clinical trials:* clinical trials are prospective, experimental studies which provide the most rigorous evidence of causality.

## 1.5   How to Quantify Variables

How do we test a hypothesis? First of all, we must set up the hypothesis in a *quantitative* manner. Our criterion measure must be a number of some sort, e.g., how many patients died in a drug group compared to how many of the patients died who did not receive the drug, or what is the mean blood pressure of patients on a certain antihypertensive drug compared to the mean blood pressure of patients not on this drug. Sometimes variables are difficult to quantify. For instance, if you are evaluating the quality of care in a clinic in one hospital compared to the clinic of another hospital, it may sometimes be difficult to find a quantitative measure that is representative of quality of care, but nevertheless, it can be done, and it must be done if one is to test the hypothesis.

There are two types of data that we can deal with: *discrete or categorical variables and continuous variables.* Continuous variables theoretically can assume an infinite number of values between any two fixed points. For example weight is a continuous variable, as is blood pressure, time, intelligence and in general variables in which measurements can be taken. Discrete variables (or categorical variables) are variables which can only assume certain fixed numerical values. For instance, sex is a discrete variable. You may code it as 1 = male, 2 = female, but an individual cannot have a score of 1.5 on sex (at least not theoretically). Discrete variables generally refer to counting, such as the number of patients in a given group who live, the number of people with a certain disease, and so on. In Section 3 we will consider a technique for testing a hypothesis where the variable is a discrete one, and subsequently, we will discuss some aspects of continuous variables, but first we will discuss the general concepts of hypothesis testing.

## 1.6   The Null Hypothesis

*The hypothesis we test statistically is called the null hypothesis.* Let us take a conceptually simple example. Suppose we are testing the efficacy of a new drug on patients with myocardial infarction (heart attack). We divide the patients into two groups: drug and no drug, according to good design procedures, and use as our criterion measure, mortality in the two groups. It is our hope that the drug lowers mortality, but to test the hypothesis statistically, we have to set it up in a sort of backward way. We say our hypothesis is that the drug makes no difference, and what we hope to do is to reject the "no difference" hypothesis, based on evidence from our sample of patients. This is known as the *null hypothesis*. We specify our test hypothesis as follows:

$H_0$ (null hypothesis):  death rate in group treated with drug A =
                             death rate in group treated with drug B
     This is equivalent to:

$H_0$ : (death rate in group A) - (death rate in group B) = 0

We test this against an *alternate hypothesis,* known as $H_A$, that the difference in death rates between the two groups *does not* equal 0.

We then gather data and note the *observed* difference in mortality between group A and group B. If this observed difference is sufficiently greater than zero difference, we reject the null hypothesis. If we reject the null hypothesis of no difference, we accept the *alternate hypothesis* which is that the drug does make a difference.

When you test a hypothesis this is the type of reasoning you use:

1. I will assume the hypothesis that there is no difference is true;
2. I will then collect the data and observe the difference between the two groups;
3. If the null hypothesis is true, how likely is it that by chance alone I would get results such as these.
4. If it is not likely that these results could arise by chance under the assumption the null hypothesis is true, then I will conclude it is false, and I will accept the alternate hypothesis."

## 1.7   Why Do We Test the Null Hypothesis?

Suppose we believe that drug A is better than drug B in preventing death from a heart attack.  Why don't we test that belief directly and see which drug is better, rather than testing the hypothesis that drug A is *equal* to drug B?  The reason is that there are an infinite number of ways in which drug A can be better than drug B, and so we would have to test an infinite number of hypotheses.  If drug A causes 10% fewer deaths than drug B, it is better.  So, first we would have to see if drug A causes 10% fewer deaths.  If it doesn't cause 10% fewer deaths, but if it causes 9% fewer deaths it is also better.  Then we would have to test whether our observations are consistent with a 9% difference in mortality between the two drugs.  Then we would have to test whether there is an 8% difference, and so on.  [Note:  each such hypothesis would be set up as a null hypothesis in the following form:  Drug A - Drug B mortality = 10% or equivalently;  (Drug A - Drug B mortality) - (10%) = 0; (Drug A - Drug B mortality - (9%) = 0; (Drug A - Drug B mortality - (8%) = 0, etc.]  On the other hand, when we test the null hypothesis of no difference, we only have to test one value: a 0% difference, and we ask the question whether our observations are consistent with the hypothesis that there is *no* difference in mortality between the two drugs.  If the observations are consistent with a null difference, then we cannot state that one drug is better than the other.  If it is unlikely that they are consistent with a null difference, then we can reject that hypothesis and conclude there is a difference.

A common source of confusion arises when the investigator really wishes to show that one treatment is as good as another (in contrast to the above example, where the investigator in her heart of hearts really believes that one drug is better.)  For example in the emergency room, a quicker procedure may have been devised and the investigator believes it may be as good as the standard procedure which takes a long time.  The temptation in such a situation is to "prove the null hypothesis".  *But it is impossible to "prove" the null hypothesis.*  All statistical tests can do is reject the null hypothesis or fail to reject it.  We do not prove your hypothesis by gathering affirmative or supportive evidence, because no matter how many times we did the experiment and found a difference close to zero, we could never be assured that the next time we did such an experiment, we would not find a huge difference that was nowhere near zero. It is like the example of the white swans discussed earlier: no matter how many white swans we see, we cannot prove that all swans are white, because the next sighting might be a black swan. Rather, we try to falsify or reject our assertion of no difference, and if the assertion of zero difference withstands our attempt at refutation, it survives as a hypothesis in which we continue to have belief. Failure to reject it does not mean we have proven that there is really no difference. It simply means that the evidence we have "is consistent with" the null hypothesis. The results we obtained, could have arisen by chance alone if the null hypothesis were true. (Perhaps the design of our study was not appropriate. Perhaps we did not have enough patients).

So what can one do if one really wants to show that two treatments are equivalent? *One can design a study that is large enough to detect a small difference if there really is one.* If the study has the power (meaning a high likelihood) to detect a difference which is very, very, very small, and one fails to detect it, then one can say with a high degree of confidence, that one can't find a meaningful difference between the two treatments. It is impossible to have a study with sufficient power to detect a 0% difference. As the difference one wishes to detect approaches zero, the number of subjects necessary for a given power approaches infinity. The relationships among significance level, power and sample size are discussed more fully in Section 5.

## 1.8  Types of Errors

The important point is that *we can never be certain* that we are right in either accepting or rejecting a hypothesis. In fact, we run the risk of making one of two kinds of errors: we can reject the null or test hypothesis incorrectly, i.e., we can conclude that the drug does reduce mortality when in actual fact it has no effect. This is known as a *type I error*. Or we can fail to reject the null or test hypothesis, incorrectly, i.e., we can conclude that the drug does not have an effect, when in fact it does reduce mortality. This is known as a *type II error*. Each of these errors caries with it certain consequences. In some cases a type I error may be more serious, in other cases a type II error may be more serious. These points are illustrated in Figure 1.2.

**Null Hypothesis ($H_0$):** *Drug has no effect* - No difference in mortality between patients using drug and patients not using drug.

**Alternate Hypothesis ($H_A$):** *Drug has effect* - Reduces mortality.

Figure 1.2

TRUE STATE OF NATURE

| | | DRUG HAS NO EFFECT; $H_O$ TRUE | DRUG HAS EFFECT; $H_O$ FALSE, $H_A$ TRUE |
|---|---|---|---|
| DECISION ON BASIS OF SAMPLE | DO NOT REJECT $H_O$ No Effect | NO ERROR | TYPE II ERROR |
| | REJECT $H_O$ (Accept $H_A$) Effect | TYPE I ERROR | NO ERROR |

If we don't reject $H_O$ we conclude there is no relationship between drug and mortality. If we do reject $H_O$ and accept $H_A$ we conclude there is a relationship between drug and mortality.

**Actions to be Taken Based on Decision:**
1.  If we believe the null hypothesis (i.e., fail to reject it) we will not use the drug.

    *Consequences of **wrong** decision:* Type II error. If we believe $H_O$ incorrectly, since in reality the drug is beneficial, by withholding it, we will allow patients to die who might otherwise have lived.

2.  If we reject null hypothesis in favor of the alternate hypothesis we will use the drug.

    *Consequences of **wrong** decision:* Type I error. If we have rejected the null hypothesis incorrectly, we will use the drug and patients don't benefit. Presuming the drug is not harmful in itself, we do not directly hurt the patients, but since we think we have found the cure, we may no longer test other drugs.

    *We can never absolutely know the "True State of Nature", but we infer it on the basis of sample evidence.*

## 1.9 Significance Level and Types of Error

We cannot eliminate the risk of making one of these kinds of errors, but we can lower the probabilities that we will make these errors. *The probability of making a type I error is known as the significance level of a statistical test.* When you read in the literature that a result was significant at the .05 level it means that in this experiment the results are such that the probability of making a type I error is less than .05. Mostly in experiments and surveys people are very concerned about having a low probability of making a type I error and often ignore the type II error. This may be a mistake since in some cases a type II error is a more serious one than a type I error. In designing a study if you aim to lower the type I error you automatically raise the type II error probability. To lower the probabilities of both the type I and type II error in a study it is necessary to increase the number of observations.

It is interesting to note that the rules of the Federal Drug Administration are set up to lower the probability of making type I errors. In order for a drug to be approved for marketing, the drug company must be able to demonstrate that it does not harm and that it is effective. Thus, many drugs are rejected because their effectiveness cannot be adequately demonstrated. The null hypothesis under test is: "This drug makes no difference." To satisfy FDA rules this hypothesis must be rejected, with the probability of making a type I error (i.e., rejecting it incorrectly) being quite low. In other words, the FDA doesn't want a lot of useless drugs on the market. Drug companies however, also give weight to guarding against type II error (i.e., avoid believing the no difference hypothesis incorrectly) so that they may market potentially beneficial drugs.

## 1.10  Consequences of Type I and Type II Errors

The relative seriousness of these errors depends on the situation. Remember, a Type I error (also known as *alpha*) means you are stating something is really there (an effect) when it actually is not, and a Type II error (also known as *beta* error) mean you are missing something that is really there. If you are looking for a cure for cancer, a type II error would be quite serious. You would miss finding useful treatments. If you are considering an expensive drug to treat a cold, clearly you would want to avoid a type I error, i.e. you would not want to make false claims for a cold remedy. It is difficult to remember the distinction between type I and II errors. Perhaps this small parable will help us.

Once there was a King who was very jealous of his Queen. He had two knights, Alpha who was very handsome, and Beta, who was very ugly. It happened that the Queen was in love with Beta. The King however, suspected the Queen was having an affair with Alpha and had him beheaded. Thus the King made both kinds of errors: he suspected a relationship (with Alpha) where there was none, and he failed to detect a relationship (with Beta) where there really was one. The Queen fled the kingdom with Beta and lived happily ever after, while the King suffered torments of guilt about his mistaken and fatal rejection of Alpha.

More on alpha, beta, power and sample size appears in Section 5. Since hypothesis testing is based on probabilities, we will first present some basic concepts of probability in Section 2.

# Section 2

# A LITTLE BIT OF PROBABILITY

*"The theory of probability is at bottom nothing but common sense reduced to calculus."*

Pierre Simon De Le Place
Theori Analytique des Probabilites (1812-1820)

## 2.1  What Is Probability?

The probability of the occurrence of an event is indicated by a number ranging from 0 to 1.  An event whose probability of occurrence is 0 is certain not to occur while an event whose probability is 1 is certain to occur.

The classical definition of probability is as follows:  if an event can occur in N mutually exclusive, equally likely ways and if $n_A$ of these outcomes have attribute A, then the probability of A, written as P(A), equals $n_A/N$.  This is an a priori definition of probability, i.e., one determines the probability of an event before it has happened.  Assume one were to toss a die and wanted to know the probability of obtaining a number divisible by three on the toss of a die.  There are six possible ways that the die can land.  Of these, there are two ways in which the number on the face of the die is divisible by three, (a 3 and a 6).  Thus, the probability of obtaining a number divisible by three on the toss of a die is 2/6 or 1/3.

In many cases, however, we are not able to enumerate all the possible ways in which an event can occur, and, therefore, we use the *relative frequency definition of probability*.  This is defined as the number of times that the event of interest has occurred divided by the total number of trials (or opportunities for the event to occur).  Since it is based on previous data, it is called the a posteriori definition of probability.

For instance, if you select at random a white, U.S., male, the probability of his dying of heart disease is .00359.  This is based on the findings that per 100,000 white American males, 359 died of coronary heart disease (estimates are from 1985, U.S. Vital and Health Statistics).[7]  When you consider the probability of a U.S. white male who is between 65 and 74 years old dying of coronary heart

13

disease, the figure rises to .015 or 1,500 deaths per 100,000 men in that age group. For black females in this age range, it is .011. The two important points are that: 1) to determine a probability, you must specify the population to which you refer, i.e., all white males, white males between 65 and 74, non-white females between 65 and 74, and so on; and, 2) the probability figures are constantly revised as new data become available.

This brings us to the notion of *expected frequency*. If the probability of an event is P and there are N trials (or opportunities for the event to occur), then we can expect that the event *will* occur N x P times. It is necessary to remember that probability "works" for large numbers. When in tossing a coin we say the probability of it landing on heads is .50, we mean that in many tosses, half the time the coin will land head. If we toss the coin ten times, we may get three heads (30%) or six heads (60%), which are a considerable departure from the 50% we expect. But if we toss the coin 200,000 times, we are very likely to be close to getting exactly 100,000 heads or 50%.

## 2.2  Combining Probabilities

There are two laws for combining probabilities that are important. First, if there are two *mutually exclusive events* (i.e., if one occurs, the other cannot), the probability of either one or the other occurring is the *sum* of their individual probabilities. Symbolically,

$$P(A \text{ or } B) = P(A) + P(B)$$

An example of this is as follows: the probability of getting either a 3 or a 4 on the toss of a die is $1/6 + 1/6 = 2/6$.

Second, if there are two *independent events*, (i.e., the occurrence of one is not related to the occurrence of the other), the joint probability of their occurring together (jointly) is the *product* of the individual probabilities. Symbolically,

$$P(A \text{ and } B) = P(A) \times P(B)$$

An example of this is the probability that on a toss of the die you will get a number that is both even and divisible by 3. This probability is equal to $1/2 \times 1/3 = 1/6$. (The only number both even and divisible by 3 is the number 6).

The joint probability law is used to test whether events are independent. If they are independent, the product of their individual probabilities should equal the joint probability. If it does not, they are not independent. It is the basis of the chi-quare test of significance which we will consider in the next section.

Let us apply these concepts to a medical example. The mortality rate for those with a heart attack in a special coronary care unit in a certain hospital is

15%.  Thus, the probability that a patient with a heart attack admitted to this coronary care unit will die is .15 and that he will survive is .85.  If two men are admitted to the coronary care unit on a particular day, let A be the event that the first man dies and let B be the event that the second man dies.  The probability that both will die is:

$$P(AandB) = P(A)\ P(B) = .15 \times .15 = .0225$$

We assume these events are independent of each other so we can multiply their probabilities.  Note however, that the probability that either one *or* the other will die from the heart attack, is *not* the sum of their probabilities because these two events are not mutually exclusive.  It is possible that both will die (i.e., both A and B can occur).

   To make this clearer, a good way to approach probability is through the use of Venn diagrams, as shown in Figure 2.1.  Venn diagrams consist of squares which represent the universe of possibilities, and circles which define the events of interest.

   In diagrams 1, 2, and 3, the space inside the square represents all N possible outcomes.  The circle marked A represents all the outcomes that constitute event A;  the circle marked B represents all the outcomes that constitute event B.  Diagram 1 illustrates two mutually exclusive events;  an outcome in circle A cannot also be in circle B.  Diagram 2 illustrates two events which can occur jointly:  an outcome in circle A can also be an outcome belonging to circle B.  The shaded area marked AB represents outcomes that are the occurrence of both A *and* B.  The diagram 3 represents two events where one (B), is a subset of the other (A):  an outcome in circle B must also be an outcome constituting event A, but the reverse is not necessarily true.

Figure 2.1

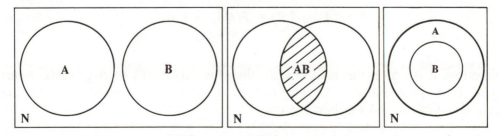

   It can be seen from diagram 2 that if we want the probability of an outcome being either A *or* B and if we add the outcomes in circle A to the outcomes in circle B, we have added in the outcomes in the shaded area twice.  Therefore, we must subtract the outcomes in the shaded area (A *and* B) also written as (AB) once to arrive at the correct answer.  Thus we get the result:

$$P(A \ or \ B) = P(A) + P(B) - P(AB)$$

## 2.3   Conditional Probability

Now let us consider the case where the chance that a particular event happens is dependent on the outcome of another event.  The probability of A, given that B has occurred is called the conditional probability of A given B, and is written symbolically as $P(A|B)$.  An illustration of this is provided by Venn diagram 2. When we speak of conditional probability, the denominator becomes all the outcomes in circle B (instead of all N possible outcomes) and the numerator consists of those outcomes which are in that part of A which also contains outcomes belonging to B.  This is the shaded area in the diagram labeled AB. If we return to our original definition of probability, we see that:

$$P(A|B) = \frac{n_{AB}}{n_B}$$

(the number of outcomes in both A *and* B, divided by the total number of outcomes in B).

   If we divide both numerator and denominator by N, the total number of *all* possible outcomes, we obtain

$$P(A|B) = \frac{n_{AB}/N}{n_B/N} = \frac{P(A \ and \ B)}{P(B)}$$

We can now derive the complete multiplicative law by multiplying both sides by P(B):

$$P(A \ and \ B) = P(A|B) \times P(B)$$

Of course, if A and B are independent, then the probability of A given B, is just equal to the probability of A (since the occurrence of B does not influence the occurrence of A) and we then see that

$$P(A \ and \ B) = P(A) \times P(B)$$

## 2.4  Summary of Probability

*Additive Law:*

$$P(A or B) = P(A) + P(B) - P(A and B)$$

if events are mutually exclusive:

$$P(A or B) = P(A) + P(B)$$

*Multiplicative Law:*

$$P(A \text{ and } B) = P(A|B) \times P(B)$$

if events are independent:

$$P(A \text{ and } B) = P(A) \times P(B)$$

*Conditional Probability:*

$$P(A|B) = \frac{P(AB)}{P(B)}$$

## 2.5  Odds and Probability

When the odds of a particular horse winning a race are said to be 4 to 1, he has a $4/5 = .80$ probability of winning.  To convert an odds statement to probability, we add the $4 + 1$ to get our denominator of 5.  If the odds of an event are 10 to 1, the probability of its happening is $10/11 = .91$;  the odds *against* the event happening are $1/11 = .09$.

## MOSTLY ABOUT STATISTICS

*"A statistician is someone who, with his head in an oven and his feet in a bucket of ice water, when asked how he feels, responds: On the average, I feel fine."*

Different statistical techniques are appropriate depending on whether the variables of interest are discrete or continuous. We will first consider the case of discrete variables and present the chi-square test and then we will discuss methods applicable to continuous variables.

### 3.1 Chi-Square for 2 x 2 Tables

The chi-square test is a statistical method to determine whether the results of an experiment may arise by chance or not. Let us, therefore consider the example of testing an anticoagulant drug on female patients with myocardial infarction. We hope the drug lowers mortality, but we set up our null hypothesis as follows:

| | |
|---|---|
| Null Hypothesis: | There is no difference in mortality between the treated group of patients and the control group. |
| Alternate Hypothesis: | The mortality in the treated group is lower than in the control group. |

(The data for our example come from a study done a long time ago and refer to a specific high risk group.[8] They are used for illustrative purposes and they do not reflect current mortality rates for people with myocardial infarction.)

We then record our data in a 2 x 2 *contingency* table in which each patient is classified as belonging to one of the 4 cells:

|         | OBSERVED FREQUENCIES | |       |
|---------|---------|---------|-------|
|         | Control | Treated |       |
| Lived   | 89      | 223     | 312   |
| Died    | 40      | 39      | 79    |
| Total   | 129     | 262     | 391   |

The mortality in the control group is $40/129 = 31\%$ and in the treated it is $39/262 = 15\%$. But could this difference have arisen by chance? We use the chi-square test to answer this question. What we are really asking is whether the two categories of classification (control vs. treated by lived vs. died) are independent of each other. If they are independent, what frequencies would we expect in each of the cells? And *how different are our observed frequencies from the expected ones?* How do we measure the size of the difference?        To determine the expected frequencies, consider the following:

|         | Control   | Treated   |       |
|---------|-----------|-----------|-------|
|         | Control   | Treated   |       |
| Lived   | a         | b         | (a + b) |
| Died    | c         | d         | (c + d) |
| Total   | (a + c)   | (b + d)   | N     |

If the categories are independent, then the probability of a patient being both a control and living is P(control) x P(lived). [Here we apply the law referred to above on the joint probability of two independent events.]

The expected frequency of an event is equal to the probability of the event times the number of trials $= N \times P$.

So the *expected number* of patients who are both controls and live is

$$N \times P(control\ and\ lived) = N \times P(control) \times P(lived)$$

$$= N\left[\frac{(a+c)}{N} \times \frac{(a+b)}{N}\right] = (a+c) \times \frac{(a+b)}{N}$$

In our case this yields the following table:

|        | Control | Treated |      |
|--------|---------|---------|------|
| Lived  | 129 x $\frac{312}{391}$ = 103 | 262 x $\frac{312}{391}$ = 209 | 312 |
| Died   | 129 x $\frac{79}{391}$ = 26 | 262 x $\frac{79}{391}$ = 53 | 79 |
| Total  | 129 | 262 | 391 |

Another way of looking at this is to say that since 80% of the treated patients in the total study lived, we would expect that 80% of the control patients and 80% of the treated patients would live. These expectations differ, as we see, from the observed frequencies noted earlier - i.e., those patients treated did, in fact, have a lower mortality than those in the control group.

Well, now that we have a table of observed frequencies and a table of expected values, how do we know just how different they are? Do they differ just by chance or is there some other factor that causes them to differ? In order to determine this, we calculate a value called chi-square (also written as $\chi^2$). This is obtained by taking the observed value in each cell, subtracting from it the expected value in each cell, squaring this difference, and dividing by the expected value for each cell. When this is done for each cell, the four resulting quantities are added together to give a number called chi-square. Symbolically this formula is as follows:

$$\frac{(O_a - e_a)^2}{e_a} + \frac{(O_b - e_b)^2}{e_b} + \frac{(O_c - e_c)^2}{e_c} + \frac{(O_d - e_d)^2}{e_d}$$

where $O$ is the observed frequency and $e$ is the expected frequency in each cell.

This number, called chi-square, is a statistic that has a known distribution. What that means in essence, is that for an infinite number of such 2 x 2 tables, chi-squares have been calculated and we thus know what the probability is of getting certain values of chi-square. Thus, when we calculate a chi-square for a particular 2 x 2 contingency table, we know how likely it is that we could have obtained a value as large as the one that we actually obtained strictly by chance, under the assumption the hypothesis of independence is the correct one, i.e., if the two categories of classification were unrelated to one another, or if the null hypothesis were true. The particular value of chi-square that we get for our example happens to be 13.94.

From our knowledge of the distribution of values of chi-square, we know that if our null hypothesis is true, i.e., if there is no difference in mortality between the control and treated group, then the probability that we get a value of chi-square as large or larger than 13.94 by chance alone is very, very low; in fact this probability is less than .005. Since it is not likely that we would get such a large value of chi-square by chance under the assumption of our null hypothesis, *it must be that it has arisen not by chance but because our null hypothesis is incorrect.* We, therefore, reject the null hypothesis at the .005 level of significance and accept the alternate hypothesis, i.e., we conclude that among women with myocardial infarction the new drug does reduce mortality. The probability of obtaining these results by chance alone is less than 5/1000 (.005). Therefore, the probability of rejecting the null hypothesis, when it is in fact true (type I error) is less than .005.

The probabilities for obtaining various values of chi-square are tabled in most standard statistics texts, so that the procedure is to calculate the value of chi-square and then look it up in the table to determine whether or not it is significant. *That value of chi-square which must be obtained from the data in order to be significant is called the critical value.* The critical value of chi-square, at the .05 level of significance for a 2 by 2 table is 3.84. This means that when we get a value of 3.84 *or greater* from a 2 x 2 table, we can say there is a significant difference between the two groups. Appendix A provides some critical values for chi-square and for other tests.

In actual usage, a correction is applied for 2 x 2 tables known as the Yates' correction and calculation is done using the formula:

$$\frac{N \left[ \mid ad - bc \mid - \dfrac{N}{2} \right]^2}{(a + b)\,(c + d)\,(a + c)\,(b + d)}$$

NOTE: $\mid ad\text{-}bc \mid$ means the absolute value of the difference between a x d and b x c. In other words, if a x d is greater than b x c, subtract bc from ad, if bc is greater than ad, subtract ad from bc. The corrected chi-square so calculated is 12.95, still well above the 3.84 required for significance.

The chi-square test should not be used if the numbers in the cells are too small. The rules of thumb are: when the total N is greater than 40, use the chi-square test with Yates' correction. When N is between 20 and 40 and the expected frequency in each of the four cells is 5 or more, use the corrected chi-square test. If the smallest expected frequency is less than 5, or if N is less than 20, use the Fisher's test.

While the chi-square test approximates the probability, the Fisher's Exact Test gives the exact probability of getting a table with values like those obtained or even more extreme. The calculations are unwieldy and will not be presented here, but may be found in the book *Statistical Methods for Rates and Proportions* by Joseph L. Fleiss. The Fisher's exact test is also usually included in most statistics programs for personal computers. The important thing is to know when the chi-square test is or is not appropriate.

## 3.2  Description of a Population:  Use of the Standard Deviation

In the case of continuous variables, as for discrete variables, we may be interested in description or in inference.  When we wish to describe a population with regard to some characteristic, we generally use the mean or average as an index of *central tendency* of the data.

Other measures of central tendency are the *median* and the *mode*.  The median is that value above which 50% of the other values lie and below which 50% of the values lie. It is the middle value or the 50th percentile.  To find the median of a set of scores we arrange them in ascending (or descending) order and locate the middle value if there are an odd number of scores, or the average between the two middle scores if there are an even number of scores.  The mode is that value which occurs with the greatest frequency.  There may be several modes in a set of scores but only one median and one mean value.  These definitions are illustrated below.  The mean is the measure of central tendency most often used in inferential statistics.

```
              Measures of Central Tendency

        set of scores              ordered
             12                        6
             12                        8
              6                       10
              8                       11   MEDIAN
             11                       12   MODE
             10                       12
             15                       15
                                 SUM 74
                                 74/7 = 10.6  MEAN
```

The true mean of the population is called $m$ and we estimate that mean from data obtained from a sample of the population.  The sample mean is called x (read as x bar). We must be careful to specify exactly the population from which we take a sample.  For instance, in the general population the average I.Q. is 100, but the average I.Q. of the population of children age 6-11 years whose fathers are college graduates is 112.[9]  Therefore, if we take a sample from either of these populations, we would be estimating a different population mean and we must specify to which population we are making inferences.

However, the mean does not provide an adequate description of a population.  What is also needed is some measure of *variability* of the data around the mean.  Two groups can have the same mean but be very different. For instance consider a hypothetical group of children each of whose individual I.Q. is 100; thus, the mean is 100.  Compare this to another group whose mean is also 100 but which includes individuals with I.Q.'s of 60 and those with I.Q.'s of 140.  Different statements must be made about these two groups:  one is composed of all average individuals; the other includes both retarded and geniuses.

The most commonly used index of variability is the *standard deviation (s.d.)*, which is a type of measure related to the average distance of the scores from their mean value. The square of the standard deviation is called *variance*. The population standard deviation is denoted by the symbol $\sigma$ (read as "sigma"). When it is calculated from *a sample*, it is written as *s.d.* and is illustrated in the example below:

| I.Q. Scores of | | Deviations from Mean | | Squared Scores for B |
|---|---|---|---|---|
| Group A | Group B | $X_i - \overline{X}_B$ | $(X_i - \overline{X}_B)^2$ | $X_B{}^2$ |
| 100 | 60 | -40 | 1600 | 3600 |
| 100 | 140 | 40 | 1600 | 19600 |
| 100 | 80 | -20 | 400 | 6400 |
| 100 | 120 | +20 | 400 | 14400 |
| Sum= $\Sigma$= 400 | $\Sigma$= 400 | $\Sigma$ = 0 | $\Sigma$= 4000 of Squared Deviations | $\Sigma$=44000 Sum of Squares |

(NOTE: The symbol "$\Sigma$" means "sum")
(NOTE: The sum of deviations from the mean, as in column 3, is always 0; that is why we sum the squared deviations, as in column 4.)

$$\overline{x}_A = mean = \frac{400}{4} = 100; \qquad \overline{x}_B = \frac{400}{4} = 100$$

$$s.d. = \sqrt{\frac{\sum of\ (each\ value - mean\ of\ group)^2}{n-1}} = \sqrt{\frac{\sum (x_i - \overline{x})^2}{n-1}}$$

$$s.d._A = \frac{0}{3} = 0;$$

(In Group A since each score is equal to the mean of 100, there are no deviations from the mean of A.)

$$s.d._B = \sqrt{\frac{4000}{3}} = \sqrt{1333} = 36.51$$

An equivalent formula for s.d. which is more suited for actual calculations is:

$$s.d. = \sqrt{\frac{\sum x_i^2 - n\overline{x}^2}{n-1}}$$

for group B we have:

$$s.d. = \sqrt{\frac{44000 - 4(100)^2}{3}} = \sqrt{\frac{44000 - 40000}{3}} = \sqrt{\frac{4000}{3}} = 36.51$$

Variance = $(s.d.)^2$

Note the mean of both groups is 100 but the standard deviation of group A is 0 while the s.d. of group B is 36.51. (We divide the squared deviations by n-1, rather than by n because we are estimating the population $\sigma$ from sample data, and dividing by n-1 gives a better estimate. The mathematical reason is complex and beyond the scope of this book.)

## 3.3  Meaning of the Standard Deviation:  The Normal Distribution

*The standard deviation is a measure of the dispersion or spread of the data.* Consider a variable like I.Q., which is normally distributed, i.e., it can be described by the familiar, bell-shaped curve where most of the values fall around the mean with decreasing number of values at either extremes. In such a case, 68 percent of the values lie within 1 standard deviation on either side of the mean, 95 percent of the values fall within 2 standard deviations of the mean, and 99 percent of the values lie within 3 standard deviations of the mean.

This is illustrated in the following Figure 3.1:

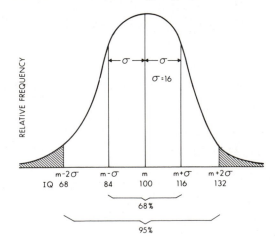

In the population at large, 95 percent of people have I.Q.'s between 68 and 132. Approximately 2.5% of people have I.Q.'s above 132 and another 2.5% of people have I.Q.'s below 68. (This is indicated by the shaded areas at the tails of the curves.)

If we are estimating from a sample and if there are a large number of observations, the standard deviation can be estimated from the *range of the data,* i.e. the difference between the smallest and the highest value. Dividing the range by 6 provides a rough estimate of the standard deviation if the distribution is normal, because 6 standard deviations (3 on either side of the mean) encompass 99% or virtually all, the data.

On an individual, clinical level, knowledge of the standard deviation is very useful in deciding whether a laboratory finding is normal, in the sense of "healthy". Generally a value that is more than two standard deviations away from the mean is suspect, and perhaps further tests need to be carried out.

For instance, suppose as a physician you are faced with an adult male who has a hematocrit reading of 39. Hematocrit is a measure of the amount of packed red cells in a measured amount of blood. A low hematocrit may imply anemia which in turn may imply a more serious condition. You also know that the average hematocrit reading for adult males is 47. Do know whether the patient with his reading of 39 is normal (in the sense of healthy) or abnormal? You need to know the standard deviation of the distribution of hematocrits in people before you can determine whether 39 is a normal value. In point of fact, the standard deviation is approximately 3.5; thus, plus or minus two standard deviations around the mean results in the range of from 40 to 54 so that 39 would be slightly low. For adult females, the mean hematocrit is 42 with a standard deviation of 2.5, so that the range of plus or minus two standard deviations away from the mean is from 37 to 47. Thus, if an adult female came to you with a hematocrit reading of 39, she would be considered in the "normal" range.

## 3.4  The Difference Between Standard Deviation and Standard Error

Often data in the literature are reported as $\bar{x} \pm$ s.d. (read as: mean + or - 1 standard deviation). Other times they are reported as $\bar{x} \pm$ s.e. (read as mean + or - 1 standard error). *Standard error* and *standard deviation* are often confused, but they serve quite different functions. To understand the concept of standard error, you must remember that the purpose of statistics is to draw inferences from samples of data to the population from which these samples came. Specifically, we are interested in estimating the true mean of a population for which we have a sample mean based on say, 25 cases. Imagine the following:

| Population<br>I.Q. scores, X | Sample means based on 25<br>people randomly selected |
|---|---|
| 110 | |
| 100 | $\overline{X}_1 = 102$ |
| 105 | |
| 98 | $\overline{X}_2 = 99$ |
| 140 | |
| | $\overline{X}_3$ |
| . | |
| . | $\overline{X}_4$ |
| 100 | 100 |

m = mean of all        $m_{\overline{X}}$ = m
    the X's        mean of the means is m,
                   the population mean

$\sigma$ = population        $\dfrac{\sigma}{\sqrt{n}}$        = standard deviation of the
    standard        distribution of the X's called
    deviation        the <u>standard error of the mean</u> = $\sigma_{\overline{X}}$

There is a population of I.Q. scores, whose mean is 100 and its standard deviation is 16. Now imagine that we draw a sample of 25 people at random from that population and calculate the sample mean $x$. This sample mean happens to be 102. If we took another sample of 25 individuals we would probably get a slightly different sample mean, for example 99. Suppose we did this repeatedly an infinite (or a very large) number of times, each time throwing the sample we just drew back into the population pool from which we would sample 25 people again. We would then have a very large number of such sample means. These sample means would form a normal distribution. Some of them would be very close to the true population mean of 100, and some would be at either end of this "distribution of means" as in Figure 3.2.

This distribution of sample means would have its own standard deviation, that is, a measure of the spread of the data around the mean of the data. In this case, the data are sample means rather than individual values. The standard deviation of this distribution of means is called *the standard error of the mean*.

It should be pointed out that this distribution of means, which is also called the sampling distribution of means, is a theoretical construct. Obviously, we don't go around measuring samples of the population to construct such a distribution. Usually, in fact, we just take *one sample of 25* people and imagine what this distribution might be. However, due to certain mathematical derivations we know a lot about this theoretical distribution of population means and therefore we can draw important inferences based on just one sample mean. What we do know is that the distribution of means is a normal distribution, that its mean is the same as the population mean of the individual values, i.e. *the mean of the means is m,* and that its standard deviation is equal to the standard deviation of the original individual values divided by the square root of the number of people in the sample.

*Standard error of the mean* =

$$\sigma_{\bar{x}} = \frac{\sigma}{\sqrt{n}}$$

In this case it would be:

$$\frac{16}{\sqrt{25}} = \frac{16}{5} = 3.2$$

The distribution of means would look as shown in Figure 3.2.

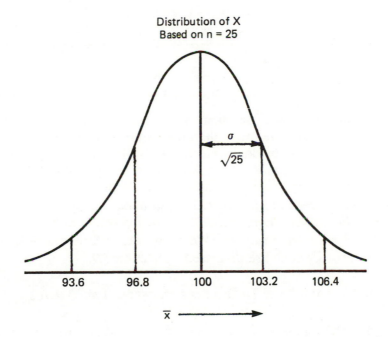

Distribution of X
Based on n = 25

$\sigma$
$\sqrt{25}$

93.6      96.8      100      103.2      106.4

$\bar{x}$ ⟶

Please note that when we talk about population values, which we usually don't know but are trying to estimate, we refer to the mean as m and the standard deviation as $\sigma$. When we talk about values calculated from samples, we refer to the mean as $\bar{x}$ and the standard deviation as s.d. and the standard error as s.e.

Now imagine that we have a distribution of means based on samples of 64 individuals. The mean of these means is also m, but its dispersion, or standard error, is smaller. It is $16\sqrt{64} = 16/8 = 2$. This is illustrated in Figure

3.3.

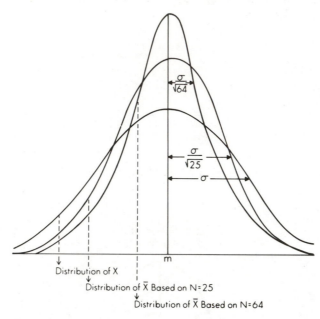

Distribution of X

Distribution of X̄ Based on N=25

Distribution of X̄ Based on N=64

It is easily seen that if we take a sample of 25 individuals their mean is likely to be closer to the true mean than the value of a single individual and if we draw a sample of 64 individuals their mean is likely to be even closer to the true mean than was the mean we obtained from the sample of 25. Thus, the larger the sample size, the better is our estimate of the true population mean.

*The standard deviation is used to tell you about the dispersion or variability of the scores. The standard error is used to draw inferences about the population mean from which we have a sample.* We draw such inferences by constructing Confidence Intervals, which are discussed in Section 3.9.

## 3.5  Standard Error of the Differences Between Two Means

This concept is analogous to the concept of standard error of the mean. The standard error of the differences between two means is the standard deviation of a theoretical distribution of differences between two means. Imagine a group of men and a group of women each of whom have an I.Q. measurement. Suppose we take a sample of 64 men and a sample of 64 women, calculate the mean I.Q.'s of these two samples and obtain their differences. If we were to do this an infinite number of times, we would get a *distribution of differences* between sample means of two groups of 64 each. These difference scores would be normally distributed; their mean would be the true average difference between the populations of men and women (which we are trying to infer from the samples); and the standard deviation of this distribution is called the *standard error of the differences between two means.*

The standard error of the difference between two means of population x and y is given by the formula:

$$\sigma_{\bar{x}-\bar{y}} = \sqrt{\frac{\sigma_x^2}{n_x} + \frac{\sigma_y^2}{n_y}}$$

where $\sigma_x^2$ is the variance of population X and $\sigma_y^2$ is the variance of population Y; $n_x$ is the number of cases in the sample from population x and $n_y$ is the number of cases from the sample from population y.

In some cases we know or assume that the variances of the two populations are equal to each other and that the variances which we calculate from the samples we have drawn are both estimates of a common variance. In such a situation, we would want to pool these estimates to get a better estimate of the common variance. We denote this *pooled estimate* as $s^2_{pooled} = s_p^2$ and we calculate the standard error of the difference between means as:

$$s.e._{\bar{x}-\bar{y}} = \sqrt{s_p^2 \left( \frac{1}{n_x} + \frac{1}{n_y} \right)} = s_p \sqrt{\frac{1}{n_x} + \frac{1}{n_y}}$$

We calculate $s^2_p$ from sample data :

$$s^2_p = \frac{(n_x-1)s_x^2 + (n_y-1)s_y^2}{n_x + n_y - 2}$$

This is the equivalent to:

$$s_p^2 = \frac{\sum(x_i-\bar{x})^2 + \sum(y_i-\bar{y})^2}{n_x+n_y-2}$$

Since in practice we will always be calculating our values from sample data, we will henceforth use the symbology appropriate to that.

### 3.6  Z Scores and the Standardized Normal Distribution

The standardized normal distribution is one whose mean = 0, standard deviation = 1 and the total area under the curve = 1.

The standard normal distribution looks like Figure 3.4

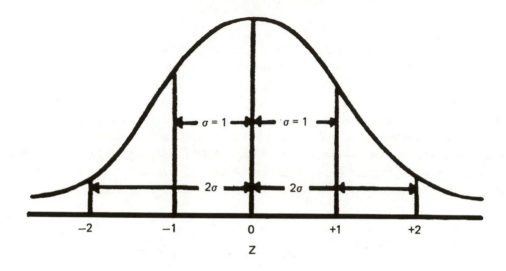

On the abscissa, instead of $x$ we have a transformation of $x$ called the standard score, Z.  Z is derived from $x$ by the following:

$$Z = \frac{\bar{x} - m}{\sigma}$$

Thus, the Z score really tells you how many standard deviations from the mean a particular $x$ score is.

Any distribution of a normal variable can be transformed to a distribution of Z by taking each $x$ value, subtracting from it the mean of $x$ and dividing this deviation of $x$ from its mean, by the standard deviation.  Let us look at the I.Q. distribution again in Figure 3.5.

Thus, an I.Q. score of 131 is equivalent to a Z score of 1.96 (i.e., it is 1.96, or nearly 2, standard deviations above the mean I.Q.).

$$Z = \frac{131 - 100}{16} = 1.96$$

Figure 3.5

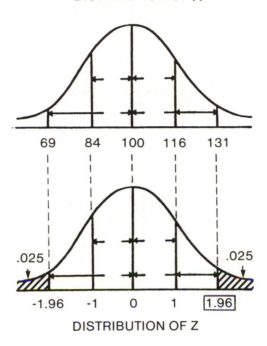

DISTRIBUTION OF X

DISTRIBUTION OF Z

One of the nice things about the Z distribution is that the probability of a value being anywhere between two points is equal to the area under the curve between those two points. (Accept this on faith). It happens that the area to the right of 1.96 corresponds to a probability of .025 or 2.5% of the total curve. Since the curve is symmetrical, the probability of Z being to the left of -1.96 is also .025. Invoking the additive law of probability (Section 2.2), the probability of a Z being *either* to the left of -1.96 *or* to the right of +1.96 is .025 + .025 = .05. Transforming back up to *x*, we can say that the probability of someone having an I.Q. outside of 1.96 standard deviations away from the mean (i.e. above 131 or below 69) is .05, or only 5% of the population have values that extreme. (Commonly, the Z value of 1.96 is rounded off to   2 standard deviations from the mean as corresponding to the cutoff points beyond which lies 5% of the curve, but the accurate value is 1.96.)

A very important use of Z derives from the fact that we can also convert a sample mean (rather than just a single individual value) to a Z score.

$$Z = \frac{\bar{x} - m}{\sigma_{\bar{x}}}$$

The numerator now is the distance of the sample mean from the population mean and the denominator is the standard deviation of the distribution of means which is the *standard error of the mean*. This is illustrated in Figure 3.6, where we are considering means based on 25 cases each. The s.e. is $16/\sqrt{25} = 16/5 = 3.2$

Figure 3.6

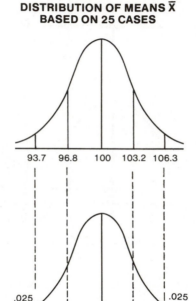

**DISTRIBUTION OF MEANS X̄
BASED ON 25 CASES**

DISTRIBUTION OF Z

Now we can see that a sample mean of 106.3 corresponds to a Z score of 1.96.

$$Z = \frac{106.3 - 100}{3.2} = 1.96$$

We can now say that the probability that the *mean* I.Q. *of a group of 25 people* is greater than 106.3 is .025. The probability that such a mean is less than 93.7 is also .025.

A Z score can also be calculated for the *difference between two means*.

$$Z = \frac{(\bar{x}_A - \bar{x}_B) - (m_A - m_B)}{\sigma_{\bar{x}_A - \bar{x}_B}}$$

But $m_A$-$m_B$ is commonly hypothesized to be 0 so the formula becomes:

$$Z = \frac{\bar{x}_A - \bar{x}_B}{\sigma_{\bar{x}_A - \bar{x}_B}}$$

You can see that a *Z score in general is a distance between some value and its mean divided by an appropriate standard error.*

This becomes very useful later on when we talk about confidence intervals in Sections 3.9-3.13.

## 3.7  The t Statistic

Suppose we are interested in sample means and we want to calculate a Z score. We don't know what the population standard deviation is, but if our samples are very large, we can get a good estimate of $\sigma$ by calculating the standard deviation, s.d., from our sample, and then getting the standard error as usual by: s.e. = s.d./$\sqrt{n}$. But often our sample is not large enough. We can still get a standardized score by calculating a value called "t".

$$t = \frac{\bar{x} - m}{s.e._{\bar{x}}}$$

It looks just like Z; the only difference is that we calculate it from the sample and it is a small sample.

We can obtain the probability of getting certain t values similarly to the way we obtained probabilities of Z values - from an appropriate table. But it happens, that while the t distribution looks like a normal Z distribution, it is just a little different, thereby giving slightly different probabilities. In fact there are many t distributions (not just one, like for Z). There is a different t distribution for each different sample size. (More will be explained about this later in Section 3.10).

In our example, where we have a mean based on 25 cases, we would need a t value of 2.06  to correspond to a probability of .025 (instead of the 1.96 for the Z distribution).  Translating this back to the scale of sample means, if our standard error were 3.2, then the probability would be .025 that we would get a sample mean as large as 106.6 (which is 2.06 times 3.2), rather than 106.3 (which is 1.96 times 3.2) as in the Z distribution.  This may seem like nit-picking, since the differences are so small. In fact, as the sample size approaches infinity, the t distribution becomes exactly like the Z distribution, but, the differences between Z and t get larger as the sample size gets smaller, and it is always safe to use the t distribution.  For example, for a mean based on 5 cases, the t value would be 2.78 instead of the Z of 1.96.  Some t values are tabled in Appendix A.  More detailed tables are in standard statistics books.

## 3.8    Sample Values and Population Values Revisited

All this going back and forth between sample values and population values may
be confusing.  Here are the points to remember:
1.  We are always interested in estimating population values from
    samples.
2.  Some of the formulas and terms we use, we apply to population
    values as if we knew them. We of course, don't know them, but if we
    have very large samples, we can estimate them quite well from our
    sample data.
3.  For practical purposes, we will generally use and refer to techniques
    appropriate for small samples, since that is more common and safer,
    (i.e. it doesn't hurt even if we have large samples).

## 3.9  A Question of Confidence

A confidence interval establishes a range and specifies the probability of the true
population mean being within that range.  For instance, a 95% confidence
interval (approximately) is set up by taking the sample mean, x plus or minus *two
standard errors of the mean*.
95% confidence interval:

$$\bar{x} \pm 2 \; s.e. = \bar{x} \pm 2\left(\frac{s.d.}{\sqrt{n}}\right)$$

Thus, if we took a random sample of 64 applicants to the Albert Einstein
College of Medicine and found their mean I.Q. to be 125, say, (a fictitious
figure) we might like to set up a 95% confidence interval to infer what the true
mean of the population of applicants really is.  We would phrase this as follows:

"the probability is .95 that the true mean I.Q. of Einstein Medical School
applicants lies within $125 \pm 2$ s.e."

For the purposes of this example, assume that the standard deviation is
16.  (This is not a particularly good assumption since the I.Q. variability of
medical school applicants is considerably less than the variability of I.Q. in the
population in general.)  Under this assumption, we arrive at the following range:

$$125 \pm \frac{2(16)}{\sqrt{64}} = 125 \pm \frac{2(16)}{8} = 125 \pm 4 = 121 - 129$$

Our statement now is as follows: "The probability is approximately .95 that the true mean I.Q. of Einstein Medical School applicants lies within the range 121-129."

A 99% confidence interval is approximately the sample mean $\pm$ 3 s.e. In our example this interval would be:

$$125 \pm 3 \left[ \frac{(16)}{\sqrt{64}} \right] = 125 \pm 6 = 119-131$$

We would then be able to say: "The probability is approximately .99 that the true mean I.Q. of Einstein Medical School applicants lies within the range 119-131."

The "approximately" is because to achieve .95 probability you don't multiply the s.e. by 2 exactly as we did here - we rounded it for convenience. The *exact* multiplying factor depends on how large the sample is. If the sample is very large, greater than 100, we would multiply the s.e. by 1.96 for 95% confidence intervals and by 2.58 for 99% confidence intervals. If the sample is smaller, we should look up the multiplier in tables of "t-values", which appear in many texts. These t-values are different for different "degrees of freedom," explained in Section 3.11 and 3.13, which are related to sample sizes. Some t values are shown in Appendix A. Also refer back to Section 3.7 for the meaning of t-statistics.

Note that for a given sample size we trade off degree of certainty for size of the interval. We can be more certain that our true mean lies within a wider range but if we want to pin down the range more precisely, we are less certain about it. (Figure 3.7). To achieve more precision and maintain a high probability of being correct in estimating the range, it is necessary to increase the sample size. The main point here is that when you report a sample mean as an estimate of a population mean, it is most desirable to report the confidence limits.

Figure 3.7

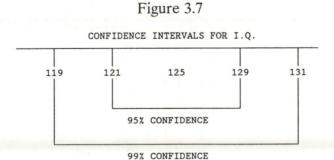

### 3.10  Confidence Limits and Confidence Intervals

Confidence limits are the outer boundaries which we calculate and about which we can say: we are 95% confident that these boundaries or limits include the true population mean. The interval between these limits is called the *confidence interval*. If we were to take a large number of samples from the population and calculate the 95% confidence limits for each of them, 95% of the intervals bound by these limits would contain the true population mean. However, 5% would not contain it. Of course, in real life, we only take one sample and construct confidence intervals from it. We can never be sure whether the interval calculated from our particular sample is one of the 5% of such intervals which do not contain the population mean. The most we can say is that we are 95% confident it does contain it. As you can see, we never know anything for sure.

   If an infinite number of independent random samples were drawn from the population of interest (with replacement), then 95% of the confidence intervals calculated from the samples (with mean: $x$, and standard error: s.e.) will encompass the true population mean, m.

   Figure 3.8 illustrates the above concepts.

## CONFIDENCE INTERVALS

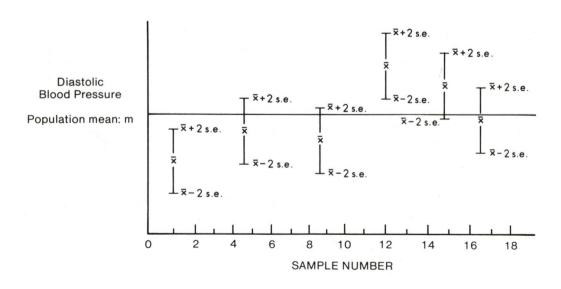

## 3.11 Degrees of Freedom

The t values which we use as the multiplier of the standard error to construct confidence intervals depend on something called the *degrees of freedom* or df, which are related to the sample size. When we have one sample, in order to find the appropriate t value to calculate the confidence limits, we enter the tables with n-1 degrees of freedom, where n is the sample size. An intuitive way to understand the concept of df is to consider that if we calculate the mean of a sample of say, 3 values, we would have the "freedom" to vary two of them any way we liked after knowing what the mean is, but the third must be fixed in order to arrive at the given mean. So we only have 2 "degrees of freedom". For example, if we know the mean of three values is 7, we can have the following sets of data:

```
value 1:       7      -50

value 2:       7      +18

value 3:       7      +53
                ─       ───
      SUM =    21       21

             x̄=7      x̄=7
```

In each case, if we know values 1 and 2, then value 3 is determined since the sum of these values must be 21 in order for the mean to be 7. We have "lost" one degree of freedom in calculating the mean.

## 3.12 Confidence Intervals for Proportions

A proportion can be considered a continuous variable. For example, in the anticoagulant study described in Section 3.1, the proportion of women in the control (placebo treated) group who survived a heart attack was found to be $89/129 = .69$. A proportion may assume values along the continuum between 0 and 1. We can construct a confidence interval around a proportion in a similar way to constructing confidence intervals around means. The 95% confidence limits for a proportion are $p \pm 1.96$ s.e.$_p$ where s.e.$_p$ is the *standard error of a proportion*. To calculate the standard error of a proportion, we must first calculate the standard deviation of a proportion and divide it by the square root of n. We define our symbology on the following page.

$s$ = *standard deviation of a proportion* = $\sqrt{pq}$

$$p = sample\ proportion = \frac{number\ of\ survivors\ in\ control\ group}{total\ number\ of\ women\ in\ control\ group}$$

$$s.e._p = \frac{\sqrt{pq}}{\sqrt{n}} = \sqrt{\frac{pq}{n}}$$

For our example of women survivors of a heart attack in the control group, the 95% confidence interval is:

$$.69 \pm 1.96 \times \sqrt{\frac{(.69) \times (.31)}{129}} = .69 \pm .08$$

And we can make the statement that we are 95% confident that the population proportion of untreated women surviving a heart attack is between .61 and .77 or 61% and 77%. (Remember this refers to the population from which our sample was drawn. We cannot generalize this to all women having a heart attack.)

For 99% confidence limits, we would multiply the standard error of a proportion by 2.58, to get the interval .59 to .80. The multiplier is the Z value that corresponds to .95 for 95% confidence limits or .99 probability for 99% confidence limits.

### 3.13 Confidence Intervals Around the Difference Between Two Means

We can construct confidence intervals around a difference between means in a similar fashion to which we constructed confidence intervals around a single mean. The 95% confidence limits around the difference between means are given by:

$$(\bar{x} - \bar{y}) \pm (t_{df, .95}) (s.e._{\bar{x} - \bar{y}})$$

In words, this is the difference between the two sample means, plus or minus an appropriate t value times the standard error of the difference; df is the degrees of freedom and .95 means we look up the t value which pertains to those degrees of freedom and to .95 probability.  The degrees of freedom when we are looking at two samples are : $n_x + n_y - 2$.  This is because we have lost one degree of freedom for each of the two means we have calculated, so our total degrees of freedom is $(n_x-1) + (n_y-1) = n_x + n_y - 2$.

As an example consider that we have a sample of 25 female and 25 male medical students.  The mean I.Q's for each sample are:

$$\bar{x}_{females} = 130, \qquad \bar{x}_{males} = 126, \qquad s_{pooled} = 12 \qquad df = 48$$

The 95% confidence interval for the mean difference between men and women is calculated as follows:

From t tables, we find that the t value for df = 48 is 2.01

$$\bar{x}_{females} - \bar{x}_{males} \pm 2.01 \times \sqrt{ s_p \left( \frac{1}{n_x} + \frac{1}{n_y} \right)} =$$

$$(130-126) \pm 2.01 \times \sqrt{12(1/25 + 1/25)} = 4 \pm 6.8$$

The interval then is -2.8 to 10.8, and we are 95% certain it includes the true mean difference between men and women.  This interval includes 0 difference, so we would have to conclude that the difference in I.Q. between men and women may be zero.

## 3.14  Comparisons Between Two Groups

A most common problem that arises is the need to compare two groups on some dimension.  We may wish to determine, for instance, whether (a) administering a certain drug lowers blood pressure, or (b) drug A is more effective than drug B in lowering blood sugar levels or (c) teaching 1st grade children to read by Method I produces higher reading achievement scores at the end of the year than teaching them to read by Method II.

## 3.15  Z-Test for Comparing Two Proportions

As an example we reproduce here the table in Section 3.1 showing data from a study on anticoagulant therapy.

|  | OBSERVED FREQUENCIES | | |
|  | Control | Treated | |
| Lived | 89 | 223 | 312 |
| Died | 40 | 39 | 79 |
| Total | 129 | 262 | 391 |

If we wish to test whether the proportion of women surviving a heart attack in the treated group differs from the proportion surviving in the control group we set up our null hypothesis as:

$H_o$:    $P_1 = P_2$ or $P_1-P_2 = 0$          $P_1$ =  proportion surviving in treated population

$P_2$ =  proportion surviving in control population

$H_A$:    $P_1-P_2 \neq 0$    (The difference does not equal 0)

We calculate:

$$Z = \frac{P_1-P_2}{s.e._{P_1-P_2}}$$

$$P_1 = \frac{223}{262} = .85 \qquad q_1 = 1-P_1 = .15 \qquad n_1 = 262$$

$$P_2 = \frac{89}{262} = .69 \qquad q_2 = 1-P_2 = .31 \qquad n_2 = 129$$

Thus the numerator of Z = .85 - .69 = .16
The denominator = *standard error of the difference between two proportions* =

$$s.e._{(P_1-P_2)} = \sqrt{\hat{p}\hat{q}\left(\frac{1}{n_1} + \frac{1}{n_2}\right)}$$

where $\hat{p}$ and $\hat{q}$ are pooled estimates based on both treated and control group data. We calculate it as follows:

$$\hat{p} = \frac{n_1 p_1 + n_2 p_2}{n_1 + n_2} = \frac{number\ of\ survivors\ in\ treated\ +\ control}{total\ number\ of\ patients\ in\ treated\ +\ control}$$

$$= \frac{262(.85) + 129(.69)}{262 + 129} = \frac{223 + 89}{391} = .80$$

$$\hat{q} = 1 - \hat{p} = 1 - .80 = .20$$

$$s.e._{(p_1 - p_2)} = \sqrt{(.80)\ (.20) \left( \frac{1}{262} + \frac{1}{129} \right)} = .043$$

$$Z = \frac{.85 - .69}{.043} = 3.72$$

We must now look to see if this value of Z exceeds the *critical value*. *The critical value is the minimum value of the test statistics which we must get in order to reject the null hypothesis at a given level of significance.*

The *critical value of* Z which we need to reject $H_o$ at the .05 level of significance is 1.96. The value we obtained is 3.74. This is clearly a large enough Z to reject $H_o$ at the .01 level at least. The critical value for Z to reject $H_o$ at the .01 level is 2.58.

Note that we came to the same conclusion using the chi-square test in Section 3.1. In fact $Z^2 = \chi^2 = (3.74)^2 = 13.99$ and the uncorrected chi-square we calculated was 13.94 (the difference is due to rounding errors). Of course the critical values of $\chi^2$ and Z have to be looked up in their appropriate tables. Some values appear in Appendix A.

### 3.16  t-Test for the Difference Between Means of Two Independent Groups:  Principles

When we wanted to compare two groups on some measure that was a discrete or categorical variable, like mortality in two groups, we used the chi-square test, described in Section 3.1. Or we could use a test between proportions as described in Section 3.15. We will now discuss a method of comparing two groups when the measure of interest is a continuous variable.

Let us take as an example the comparison of the ages at first pregnancy of two groups of women: those who are lawyers and those who are para-legals. Such a study might be of sociological interest, or it might be of interest to law firms, or perhaps to a baby foods company which is seeking to focus its advertising strategy more effectively.

Assuming we have taken proper samples of each group, we now have two sets of values: the ages of the lawyers (Group A) and the ages of the para-legals (Group B), and we have a mean age for each sample.

We set up our null hypothesis as follows:

$H_o$:    "The mean age of the population of lawyers from which we have drawn sample A is the same as the mean age of the population of para-legals from which we have drawn sample B."

Our alternate hypothesis is:

$H_A$:    "The mean ages of the two populations we have sampled are different.

In essence then, *we have drawn samples on the basis of which we will make inferences about the populations from which they came.* We are subject to the same kinds of type I and type II errors we discussed before.

The general approach is as follows. We know there is variability of the scores in group A around the mean for group A and within group B around the mean for group B, simply because even within a given population, people vary. What we want to find is whether the variability between the 2 sample means around the grand mean of all the scores is greater than the variability of the ages within the groups around their own means. If there is as much variability within the groups as between the groups, then they probably come from the same population.

The appropriate test here is the t-test. We calculate a value known as t, which is equal to the difference between the two sample means divided by an appropriate standard error. The appropriate standard error is called the standard error of the difference between two means and is written as:

$$s.e._{\bar{x}_1 - \bar{x}_2}$$

The distribution of t has been tabulated and from the tables we can obtain the probability of getting a value of t as large as the one we actually obtained under the assumption that our null hypothesis (of no difference between means) is true. If this probability is small (i.e., if it is unlikely that by chance alone we would get a value of t that large if the null hypothesis were true) we would reject the null hypothesis and accept the alternate hypothesis that there really is a difference between the means of the populations from which we have drawn the two samples.

## 3.17  How to Do a t-Test - An Example

Although t-tests can be easily performed on most personal computers, an example of the calculations and interpretation is given below. This statistical test is performed to compare the means of two groups under the assumption that both samples are random, independent and come from normally distributed populations with unknown but equal variances.

*Null Hypothesis*:  $m_A = m_B$, or the equivalent:  $m_A - m_B = 0$

*Alternate Hypothesis*:  $m_A \neq m_B$ or the equivalent:  $m_A - m_B \neq 0$

[NOTE:  When the alternate hypothesis does not specify the direction of the difference (by stating for instance that $m_A$ is greater than $m_B$) but simply says the difference *does not equal 0*, it is called a two-tailed test. When the direction of the difference is specified, it is called a one-tailed test. More on this topic appears in Section 5.4.]

$$t = \frac{(\bar{x}_A - \bar{x}_B)}{s_{\bar{x}_A - \bar{x}_B}}$$

| Ages of Sample A $x_i$ | $(x_i - \bar{x}_A)$ | $(x_i - \bar{x}_A)^2$ | Ages of Sample B $x_i$ | $(x_i - \bar{x}_B)$ | $(x_i - \bar{x}_B)^2$ |
|---|---|---|---|---|---|
| 28 | -3 | 9 | 24 | 2.4 | 5.76 |
| 30 | -1 | 1 | 25 | 3.4 | 11.56 |
| 27 | -4 | 16 | 20 | -1.6 | 2.56 |
| 32 | 1 | 1 | 18 | -3.6 | 12.96 |
| 34 | 3 | 9 | 21 | .6 | 0.36 |
| 36 | 5 | 25 | $\Sigma = 108$ | $\Sigma = 0$ | $\Sigma = 33.20$ |
| 30 | -1 | 1 | | | |
| $\Sigma = 217$ | $\Sigma = 0$ | $\Sigma = 62$ | | | |

$$Mean_A = \bar{x}_A = \frac{\Sigma x_i}{n} = \frac{217}{7} = 31; \quad Mean_B = \bar{x}_B = \frac{\Sigma x_i}{n} = \frac{108}{5} = 21.6$$

(The subscript "i" refers to the ith score and is a convention used to indicate that we sum over all the scores.)

The numerator of t is the difference between the two means:  $31 - 21.6 = 9.4$
To get the denominator of t we need to calculate the standard error of the difference between means, which we do as follows:

First we get the pooled estimate of the standard deviation.  We calculate:

$$s_p = \sqrt{\frac{\Sigma(x_i-\bar{x}_A)^2 + \Sigma(x_i-\bar{x}_B)^2}{n_A + n_B - 2}} = \sqrt{\frac{62 + 33.20}{7 + 5 - 2}} = \sqrt{\frac{95.20}{10}} = \sqrt{9.52} = 3.09$$

$$s_{\bar{x}_A-\bar{x}_B} = s_p\sqrt{\frac{1}{n_A} + \frac{1}{n_B}} = 3.09\sqrt{\frac{1}{7} + \frac{1}{5}} = 3.09\sqrt{.3428} = 3.09 \times .5854 = 1.81$$

$$t = \frac{\bar{x}_A-\bar{x}_B}{s_{\bar{x}_A-\bar{x}_B}} = \frac{9.4}{1.81} = 5.19$$

This t is significant at the .001 level, which means that you would get a value of t as high as this one or higher only 1 time out of a thousand by chance if the null hypothesis were true.  So we reject the null hypothesis of no difference, accept the alternate hypothesis, and conclude that the lawyers are older at first pregnancy than the para-legals.

## 3.18  Matched Pair t-Test

If you have a situation where the scores in one group correlate with the scores in the other group, you cannot use the regular t-test since that assumes the two groups are independent.  This situation arises when you take two measures on the same individual.  For instance, suppose group A represents reading scores of a group of children taken at time 1.  These children have then been given special instruction in reading over a period of six months and their reading achievement is again measured to see if they accomplished any gains at time 2. In such a situation you would use a matched pair t-test.

| Child | A<br>Initial<br>reading<br>scores of<br>Children | B<br>Scores<br>of same<br>children<br>after<br>6 months<br>training | d = B - A | d - d̄ | (d-d̄)2 |
|-------|------|------|------|------|------|
| (1) | 60 | 62 | 2 | 1.4 | 1.96 |
| (2) | 50 | 54 | 4 | 3.4 | 11.56 |
| (3) | 70 | 70 | 0 | -.6 | .36 |
| (4) | 80 | 78 | -2 | -2.6 | 6.76 |
| (5) | 75 | 74 | -1 | -1.6 | 2.50 |

Sum    3                0               23.20
mean difference = d̄ = 3/5 = 0.60

***Null Hypothesis***:  mean difference = 0

***Alternate Hypothesis***:  mean difference is greater than 0

$$t = \frac{\bar{d}}{s_{\bar{d}}} \; ; \qquad s_{\bar{d}} = \frac{s}{\sqrt{n}}$$

$$s = \frac{\sqrt{\Sigma(d-\bar{d})^2}}{n-1} = \sqrt{\frac{23.20}{4}} = \sqrt{5.8} = 2.41$$

$$s_{\bar{d}} = \frac{2.41}{\sqrt{5}} = \frac{2.41}{2.23} = 1.08$$

$$t = \frac{.60}{1.08} = .56$$

This t is not significant, which means that we do not reject the null hypothesis and conclude that the mean difference in reading scores could be zero; i.e., the six months reading program may not be effective. (Or it may be that the study was not large enough to detect a difference, and we have committed a beta error.)

### 3.19  When Not to Do a Lot of t-Tests - The Problem of Multiple Tests of Significance

A t-test is used for comparing the means of two groups.  When there are three or more group means to be compared, the t-test is not appropriate. To understand why, we need to invoke our knowledge of combining probabilities from Section 2.2.

Suppose you are testing the effects of three different treatments for high blood pressure.  Patients in one group receive medication A, a diuretic; patients in group B receive another medication, a beta-blocker; and patients in group C receive a placebo pill.  You want to know whether either drug is better than placebo in lowering blood pressure and if the two drugs are different from each other in their blood pressure lowering effect.

There are three comparisons that can be made: Group A vs. Group C (to see if the diuretic is better than placebo); Group B versus group C (to see if the beta blocker is better than the placebo) and Group A versus Group B (to see which of the two active drugs has more effect.  We set our significance level at .05, i.e. we are willing to be *wrong* in rejecting the null hypothesis of no difference between two means, with a probability of .05 or less (i.e. our probability of making a type I error must be no greater than .05).  Consider the following:

| Comparison | Probability of of Type I error | Probability of not making a Type I error = 1-P (Type I error) |
|---|---|---|
| 1. A vs. C | .05 | 1 - .05 = .95 |
| 2. B vs. C | .05 | 1 - .05 = .95 |
| 3. A vs. B | .05 | 1 - .05 = .95 |

The probability of *not* making a Type I error in the first comparison *and* not making it in the second comparison *and* not making it in the third comparison = $.95 \times .95 \times .95 = .86$ .  We are looking here at the *joint* occurrence of three events (the three ways of *not* committing a Type I error) and we combine these probabilities by multiplying the individual probabilities. (Remember, when we see "and" in the context of combining probabilities, we multiply, when we see "or" we add.)  So now, we know that the overall probability of *not* committing a Type I error in any of the three possible comparisons is .86.  Therefore, the probability of committing such an error is 1- the probability of not committing it, or 1-.86 = .14.  Thus, the overall probability of a Type I error would be considerably greater than the .05 we specified as desirable.  In actual fact, the numbers are a little different because the three comparisons are not independent events, since the same groups are used in more than one comparison, so combining probabilities in this situation would not involve the simple multiplication rule for the joint occurrence of independent events. However, it is close enough to illustrate the point that making multiple comparisons in the same experiment results in quite a different significance level (.14 in this example) than the one we chose (.05). When there are more than three groups to compare, the situation gets worse.

## 3.20   Analysis of Variance - Comparison Among Several Groups

The appropriate technique for analyzing continuous variables when there are three or more groups to be compared is the analysis of variance, commonly referred to as ANOVA.  An example might be comparing the blood pressure reduction effects of the three drugs.

## 3.21   Principles

The principles involved in the analysis of variance are the same as those in the t-test.  Under the null hypothesis we would have the following situation: there would be one big population and if we picked samples of a given size from that population we would have a bunch of sample means which would vary due to chance around the grand mean of the whole population.  If it turns out they vary around the grand mean more than we would expect just by chance alone, then perhaps something other than chance is operating.  Perhaps they don't all come from the same population.  Perhaps something distinguishes the groups we have picked. We would then reject the null hypothesis that all the means are equal and conclude the means are different from each other by more than just chance. Essentially, we want to know if the variability of all the groups means is substantially greater than the variability within each of the groups around their own mean.

We calculate a quantity known as the *between-groups variance*, which is the variability of the group means around the grand mean of all the data.  We calculate another quantity called the *within-groups variance*, which is the variability of the scores within each group around its own mean.  One of the assumptions of the analysis of variance is that the extent of the variability of individuals within groups is the same for each of the groups, so we can pool the estimates of the individual within group variances to obtain a more reliable estimate of overall within-groups variance.  If there is as much variability of individuals within the groups as there is variability of means between the groups, they probably come from the same population which would be consistent with the hypothesis of no true difference among means; i.e. we could not reject the null hypothesis of no difference among means.

*The ratio of the between-groups variance to the within-groups variance is known as the F ratio.* Values of the F distribution appear in tables in many statistical texts and if the obtained value from our experiment is greater than the *critical value* which is tabled, we can then reject the hypothesis of no difference.

There are different critical values of F depending on how many groups are compared and on how many scores there are in each group. To read the tables of F, one must know the two values of "degrees of freedom" (df). The df corresponding to the between-groups variance, which is the numerator of the F ratio, is equal k-1, where k is the number of groups. The df corresponding to the denominator of the F ratio, (which is the within-groups variance), is equal to k x (n-1), i.e. the number of groups times the number of scores in each group minus one. For example, if in our hypertension experiment there are 100 patients in each of the 3 drug groups, then the numerator degrees of freedom would be 3-1 = 2, and the denominator degrees of freedom would be 3 x 99 = 297. An F ratio would have to be at least 3.07 for a significance level of .05. If there were 4 groups being compared then the numerator degrees of freedom would be 3, and the critical value of F would need to be 2.68. If there are not an equal number of individuals in each group, then the denominator degrees of freedom is $(n_1-1) + (n_2-1) + (n_3-1)$.

We will not present here the actual calculations necessary to do an F test because nowadays these are rarely done by hand. There are a large number of programs available for personal computers which can perform F tests, t-tests and most other statistical analyses. However, shown below is the kind of output that can be expected from these programs. Shown are summary data from the TAIM study (Trial of Antihypertensive Interventions and Management). The TAIM Study is designed to evaluate the effect of diet and drugs, used alone or in combination with each other, to treat overweight persons with mild hypertension (high blood pressure).[10,11]

The table below shows the mean drop in blood pressure after six months of treatment with each drug, the number of people in each group, and the standard deviation of the *change* in blood pressure in each group.

| DRUG GROUP | n | Mean drop in diastolic blood pressure units after 6 months of treatment | Standard Deviation |
|---|---|---|---|
| A. Diuretic | 261 | 12.1 | 7.9 |
| B. Beta-Blocker | 264 | 13.5 | 8.2 |
| C. Placebo | 257 | 9.8 | 8.3 |

Below is a table resulting from an analysis of variance of the data from this study. It is to be interpreted as follows:

ANOVA

| Source of variation | Degrees of freedom | Sum of Squares | Mean Square | F ratio | P₂>F |
|---|---|---|---|---|---|
| Between Groups | 2 | 1776.5 | 888.2 | 13.42 | .0001 |
| Within Groups | 779 | 5256.9 | 66.2 | | |
| | 781 | | | | |

The Mean Square is the sum of squares divided by the degrees of freedom. For between-groups, it is the variation of the group means around the grand mean, while for within-groups, it is the pooled estimate of the variation of the individual scores around their respective group means. The within-groups mean square is also called the Error Mean Square. (An important point is that the square root of the Error Mean Square is the pooled estimate of the within-groups standard deviation. In this case is $\sqrt{66.2} = 8.14$. It is roughly equivalent to the average standard deviation.) F is the ratio of the between to the within mean squares; in this example it is $888.2/66.2 = 13.42$.

The F ratio is significant at the .0001 level, so we can reject the null hypothesis that *all* group means are equal. However, we do not know where the difference lies. Is group A different from group C but not from group B? We should not simply make all the pair-wise comparisons possible because of the problem of multiple comparisons discussed above. But there are ways to handle this problem. One of them is the Bonferroni procedure, described in the next Section 3.22.

### 3.22 Bonferroni Procedure: An Approach to Making Multiple Comparisons

This is one way to handle the problem of multiple comparisons. The Bonferroni procedure implies that if for example we make 5 comparisons, the probability that *none* of the five p values falls below .05 is at least 1-(5 x .05) = .75 when the null hypothesis of equal means is really true. That means that there is a probability of up to .25 that at least one p value will reach the .05 significance level by chance alone *even if the treatments really do not differ*. To get around this, we divide the chosen overall significance level by the number of two-way comparisons to be made, consider this value to be the significance level for any single comparison, and reject the null hypothesis of no difference only if it achieves this new significance level.

For example, if we want an overall significance level of .05 and we will make three comparisons between means, we would have to achieve .05/3 = .017

level in order to reject the null hypothesis and conclude there is a difference between the two means. A good deal of self-discipline is required to stick to this procedure and not declare a difference between two means as unlikely to be due to chance if the particular comparison has significance at p = .03, say, instead of .017. The Bonferroni procedure does not require a prior F test. Let us apply the Bonferroni procedure to our data.

First we compare each of the drugs to placebo. We calculate the t for the difference between means of group A vs. group C.

$$t = \frac{\bar{x}_A - \bar{x}_C}{s.e._{\bar{x}_A - \bar{x}_C}}$$

$$s.e._{\bar{x}_A - \bar{x}_C} = s_p \sqrt{\frac{1}{n_A} + \frac{1}{n_C}}$$

$$\frac{12.1 - 9.8}{8.14\sqrt{\frac{1}{261} + \frac{1}{257}}} = \frac{2.3}{.715} = 3.22$$

$$p = .0014$$

Note that we use 8.14 as s pooled. We obtained this from the analysis of variance as an estimate of the common standard deviation. The degrees of freedom to enter the t tables are 261 + 257 - 2 = 516.

It turns out that the probability of getting such a high t value by chance is .0014. We can safely say the diuretic reduces blood pressure more than the placebo. The same holds true for the comparison between the beta-blocker and placebo. Now let us compare the two drugs, B vs. A:

$$t = \frac{13.5 - 12.1}{8.14\sqrt{\frac{1}{264} + \frac{1}{261}}} = \frac{1.4}{.711} = 1.97$$

The p value corresponding to this t value is .049. It might be tempting to declare a significant difference at the .05 level, but remember the Bonferroni procedure requires that we get a p value of .017 or less for significance adjusted for multiple comparisons. The critical value of t corresponding to p=.017 is 2.39 and we only got a t of 1.97. Recently[12], there has been some questioning of the routine adjustment for multiple comparisons on the grounds that we thereby may commit more type II errors and miss important effects. In any case p levels should be reported so that the informed reader may evaluate the evidence.

### 3.23  Analysis of Variance When There Are Two Independent Variables - The Two-Factor ANOVA

The example above is referred to as the one-way ANOVA because you can divide all the scores in one way only, by the drug group to which patients were assigned. The drug group is called a "factor" and this factor has 3 levels, meaning there are three categories of drug. There may, however, be another factor which classifies individuals, and in that case we would have a two-way, or a two factor, ANOVA. In the experiment we used as an example, patients were assigned to one of the three drugs noted above, as well as to one of three diet regimens (weight reduction, salt restriction, or no change from their usual diet, which is analogous to a placebo diet condition). The diagram below illustrates this two-factor design, and the mean drop in blood pressure in each group, as well as the numbers of cases in each group which are shown in parenthesis.

|  | DIET | | | |
| --- | --- | --- | --- | --- |
| DRUG | Usual | Weight Reduction | Salt Restriction | Total |
| Diuretic | 10.2 (87) | 14.5 (86) | 11.6 (88) | 12.1 (261) |
| Beta-Blocker | 12.8 (86) | 15.2 (88) | 12.6 (90) | 13.5 (264) |
| Placebo | 8.7 (89) | 10.8 (89) | 10.1 (79) | 9.8 (257) |
| Total | 10.5 (262) | 13.5 (263) | 11.5 (257) | |

Now we are interested in comparing the three means which represent change in blood pressure in the drug groups, the three means which represent changes in the diet groups, and the interaction between drug and diet. We now explain the concept of interaction.

## 3.24  Interaction Between Two Independent Variables

*Interaction* between two independent variables refers to differences in the effect of one variable depending on the level of the second variable.  For example, maybe one drug produces better effects when combined with a weight reduction diet than when combined with a salt restricted diet.  There may not be a significant effect of that drug when all diet groups are lumped together but if we look at the effects separately for each diet group we may discover an interaction between the two factors:  diet and drug.

The diagrams below illustrate the concept of interaction effects.  WR means weight reduction and SR means salt restriction.

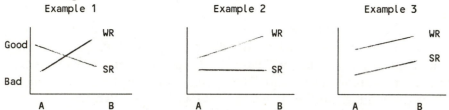

In example 1 drug B is better than drug A in those under weight reduction but in those under salt restriction Drug A is better than Drug B.  If we just compared the average for drug A, combining diets, with the average for drug B, we would have to say there is no difference between drug A and drug B, but if we look at the two diets separately, we see quite different effects of the two drugs.

In example 2, there is no difference in the two drugs for those who restrict salt, but there is less effect of drug A than drug B for those in weight reduction.

In example 3, there is no interaction;  there is an equal effect for both diets, the two lines are parallel, their slopes are the same.

## 3.25  Example of a Two-Way ANOVA

Below is a table of actual data from the TAIM study showing the results of a *two-way analysis of variance*;

Two-Way ANOVA From TAIM Data

| Source | DF | ANOVA Sum of Squares | Mean Square | F Value | Probability |
|--------|----|----|----|----|----|
| Drug Group | 2 | 1776.49 | 888.25 | 13.68 | .0001 |
| Diet Group | 2 | 1165.93 | 582.96 | 8.98 | .0001 |
| Drug x Diet | 4 | 214.50 | 53.63 | 0.83 | .509 |
| Error | 773 | 50185.46 | 64.93 | | |

Note that the error mean square here is 64.93 instead of 66.9 when we did the one-way analysis. That is because we have explained some of the error variance as being due to diet effects and interaction effects; (we have "taken out" these effects from the error variance). Thus, 64.93 represents the variance due to pure error, or the unexplained variance. Now we can use the square root of this which is 8.06 as the estimate of the common standard deviation. We explain the results as follows:

There is a significant effect of drug (p=.0001) and a significant effect of diet (p=.0001) but no interaction of drug by diet (p=.509).

We have already made pairwise comparisons among the drugs and concluded that both are better than placebo but not different from each other. We can do the same for the three diets. Their mean values are displayed below.

| Diet Group | n | Mean Drop in Diastolic Blood Pressure | Standard Deviation |
|---|---|---|---|
| Weight Reduction | 263 | 13.5 | 8.3 |
| Salt Restriction | 257 | 11.5 | 8.3 |
| Usual Diet | 262 | 10.5 | 8.0 |
| (pooled estimate of s.d. = 8.06) | | | |

If we did t-tests, we would find that weight reduction is better than usual diet (p=.0000) but salt restriction is no improvement over usual diet (p=.16).

Weight reduction when compared to salt restriction is also significantly better with p=.005 which is well below the p=.017 required by the Bonferroni procedure. (The t for this pairwise comparison is 2.83, which is above the critical value of 2.39).

## 3.26 Association and Causation - The Correlation Coefficient

A common class of problems in the accumulation and evaluation of scientific evidence is the assessment of association of two variables. Is there an association between poverty and drug addiction? Is emotional stress associated with cardiovascular disease?

In order to determine association, we must first quantify both variables. For instance, emotional stress may be quantified by using an appropriate psychological test of stress or by clearly defining, evaluating and rating on a scale, the stress factor in an individual's life situation, while hypertension (defined as a blood pressure reading) may be considered as the particular aspect of cardiovascular disease to be studied. When variables have been quantified, a measure of association needs to be calculated to determine the strength of the relationship. One of the most common measures of association is the *correlation coefficient*, r.

The correlation coefficient, r, is a number derived from the data that can vary between -1 and +1. (The method of calculation appears in Appendix B.) When r = 0 it means there is no association between the two variables. An example of this might be the correlation between blood pressure and the number of hairs on the head. When r = +1, a perfect positive correlation, it means there is a direct relationship between the two variables: an individual who has a high score on one variable, also has a high score on the other and the score on one variable can be exactly predicted from the score on the other variable. This kind of correlation exists only in deterministic models, where there is really a functional relationship. An example might be the correlation between age of a tree and the number of rings it has. A correlation coefficient of -1 indicates a perfect inverse relationship, where a high score on one variable means a low score on the other and where, as in perfect positive correlation, there is no error of measurement. Correlation coefficient between 0 and +1 and between 0 and -1 indicate varying strengths of associations.

These correlation coefficients apply when the basic relationship between the two variables is linear. Consider a group of people on each of whom we have a measurement of weight against height; we will find that we can draw a straight line through the points. There is a linear association between weight and height and the correlation coefficient would be positive but less than 1.

The following diagrams illustrate representations of various correlation coefficients (Figure 3.9).

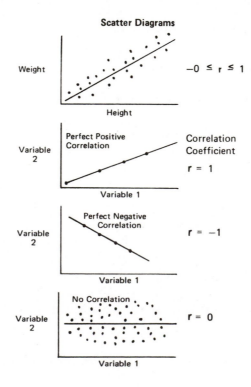

## 3.27  How High Is High?

The answer to this question depends upon the field of application as well as on many other factors.  Among psychological variables, which are difficult to measure precisely and are affected by many other variables, the correlations are generally (though not necessarily) lower than among biological variables where more accurate measure-ment is possible.  The following example may give you a feel for the orders of magnitude.  The correlations between verbal aptitude and non-verbal aptitude, as measured for Philadelphia school children, by standardized national tests, range from .44 to .71 depending on race and social class of the groups.[13]

## 3.28  Causal Pathways

If we do get a significant correlation, we then ask what situations could be responsible for it?  Some possibilities are illustrated in Figure 3.10, where we consider two variables, $Y_1$ and $Y_2$, and let $r_{12}$ represent the correlation between them.[14]  In examining Figure 5, note that only in diagrams A and F does the correlation between $Y_1$ and $Y_2$, arise due to a causal relationship between the two variables  In diagram A, $Y_2$ is the entire cause of $Y_1$ and in diagram F, $Y_2$ is a partial cause of $Y_1$.  In all of the other structural relationships the correlation between $Y_1$ and $Y_2$ arises due to common influences on both variables.  Thus, it must be stressed that *the existence of a correlation between two variables does not necessarily imply causation.*  Correlations may arise because one variable is the partial cause of another or the two correlated variables have a common cause.  Other factors such as sampling, the variation in the two populations, and so on, affect the size of the correlation coefficient also.  Thus, care must be taken in interpreting these coefficients.

Figure 3.10

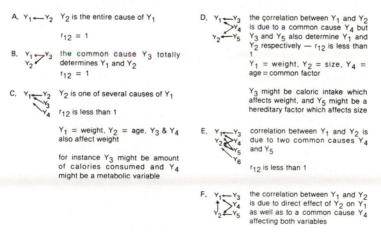

## 3.29 Regression

Note that in Figure 3.9 we have drawn lines that seem to best fit the data points. These are called *regression lines*. They have the following form: $Y = a + bX$. In the top scattergram labeled a), Y is the dependent variable weight and X, or height, is the independent variable. We say that weight is a function of height. The quantity a is the intercept. It is where the line crosses the y axis. The quantity b is the slope and it is the rate of change in Y for a unit change in X. If the slope is 0, it means we have a straight line parallel to the X axis, as in the illustration d). It also means that we cannot predict Y from a knowledge of X since there is no relationship between Y and X. If we have the situation shown in scattergrams b) or c), we know exactly how Y changes when X changes and we can perfectly predict Y from a knowledge of X with no error. In the scattergram a), we can see that as X increases Y increases but we can't predict Y perfectly because the points are scattered around the line we have drawn. We can, however, put confidence limits around our prediction, but first we must determine the form of the line we should draw through the points. We must estimate the values for the intercept and slope. This is done by finding the "best-fit line".

The line that fits the points best has the following characteristics: if we take each of the data points and calculate its vertical distance from the line and then square that distance, the sum of those squared distances will be smaller than the sum of such squared distances from any other line we might draw. This is called the *least-squares* fit. Consider the data below where Y could be a score on one test and X could be a score on another test.

|            | Score |     |
| :--------: | :---: | :-: |
| **Individual** | **X** | **Y** |
| A          | 5     | 7   |
| B          | 8     | 4   |
| C          | 15    | 8   |
| D          | 20    | 10  |
| E          | 25    | 14  |

The calculations to determine the best-fit line are shown in Appendix C. However, most statistical computer packages for personal computers provide a linear regression program that does these calculations. Figure 3.11 illustrates these points plotted in a scattergram and shows the least-squares line.

Figure 3.11

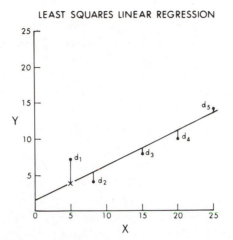

The equation for the line is: $Y = 2.76 + .40\ X$

The intercept a, is 2.76 so that the line crosses the Y axis at $Y = 2.76$. The slope is .40. For example, we can calculate a predicted Y for $X = 10$ to get

$$Y = 2.76 + (.40)(10) = 2.76 + 4 = 6.76$$

The $d_i$'s are distances from the points to the line. It is the sum of these squared distances that is smaller for this line than it would be for any other line we might draw.

The correlation coefficient for these data is .89. The square of the correlation coefficient, $r^2$, can be interpreted as the proportion of the variance in Y that is explained by X. In our example, $.89^2 = .79$; thus 79% of the variation of Y is explainable by the variable X, and 21% is unaccounted for.

### 3.30  The Connection Between Linear Regression and the Correlation Coefficient

The correlation coefficient and the slope of the linear regression line are related by the formula:

$$r = b\frac{s_x}{s_y} \qquad\qquad\qquad b = r\frac{s_y}{s_x}$$

where $s_x$ is the standard deviation of the x variable, $s_y$ is the standard deviation of the y variable, b is the slope of the line and r is the correlation coefficient.

## 3.31  Multiple Linear Regression

When we have two or more independent variables and a continuous dependent variable, we can use multiple regression analysis. The form this takes is:

$$Y = a + b_1X_1 + b_2X_2 + b_3X_3 + ....b_kX_k$$

For example, Y may be blood pressure and $X_1$ may be age, $X_2$ may be weight, $X_3$ may be family history of high blood pressure. We can have as many variables as appropriate, where the last variable is the kth variable. The $b_i$'s are *regression coefficients*. Note that family history of high blood pressure is not a continuous variable. It can either be yes or no. We call this a dichotomous variable and we can use it as any other variable in a regression equation by assigning a number to each of the two possible answers, usually by making a yes answer = 1 and a no answer = 0.

Statistical computer programs usually include multiple linear regression.

An example from the TAIM Study follows and is meant only to give you an idea of how to interpret a multiple regression equation. This analysis pertains to the group of 89 people who were assigned to a placebo drug and a weight reduction regimen. The dependent variable is change in blood pressure.

The independent variables are shown below:

| Variable | Coefficient: $b_i$ | p |
|---|---|---|
| Intercept | -15.49 | .0016 |
| Age | .077 | .359 |
| Race  1=Black<br>        0=Non-Black | 4.22 | .021 |
| Sex   1=Male<br>        0=Female | 1.50 | .390 |
| Pounds Lost | .13 | .003 |

Note: Sex is coded as 1 if male and 0 if female;  race is coded as 1 if black and 0 if non-black.  p is used to test if the coefficient is significantly different from 0.  The equation, then, is:

change in blood pressure   = -15.49 + .077(age) + 4.22(race) + 1.5(sex)
                              + .13(change in weight)

Age is not significant (p=.359) nor is sex (p=.390).  However, race is significant (p=.021) indicating that blacks were more likely than non-blacks to have a drop in blood pressure while simultaneously controlling for all the other variables in the equation. Pounds lost is also significant, indicating that the greater the weight loss, the greater was the drop in blood pressure.

## 3.32  Summary So Far

Investigation of a scientific issue often requires statistical analysis, especially where there is variability with respect to the characteristics of interest. The variability may arise from two sources: the characteristic may be inherently variable in the population and/or there may be error of measurement.

In this section we have pointed out that in order to evaluate a program or a drug, to compare two groups on some characteristic, to conduct a scientific investigation of any issue, it is necessary to quantify the variables.

Variables may be quantified as discrete or as continuous and there are appropriate statistical techniques which deal with each of these. We have considered here the chi-square test, confidence intervals, Z-test, t-test, analysis of variance, correlation and regression. We have pointed out that in hypothesis testing we are subject to two kinds of errors: the error of rejecting a hypothesis when in fact it is true, and the error of accepting a hypothesis when in fact it is false. The aim of a well-designed study is to minimize the probability of making these types of errors. Statistics will not substitute for good experimental design, but it is a necessary tool to evaluate scientific evidence obtained from well-designed studies.

Philosophically speaking, statistics is a reflection of life in two important respects: 1) As in life, we can never be certain of anything (but in statistics we can put a probability figure describing the degree of our uncertainty), and 2) All is a trade-off: in statistics, between certainty and precision, or between two kinds of error; in life, well, fill in your own trade-offs.

# Section 4

## MOSTLY ABOUT EPIDEMIOLOGY

*"Medicine to produce health has to examine disease; and music to create harmony, must investigate discord."*
Plutarch
A.D. 46-120

### 4.1 The Uses of Epidemiology

Epidemiology may be defined as the study of the distribution of health and disease in *groups of people* and the study of the factors that influence this distribution. Modern epidemiology also encompasses the evaluation of diagnostic and therapeutic modalities and the delivery of health care services. There is a progression in the scientific process (along the dimension of increasing credibility of evidence), from casual observation, to hypothesis formation, to controlled observation, to experimental studies. Figure 4.1 is a schematic representation of the uses of epidemiology. The tools used in this endeavor are in the province of epidemiology and biostatistics. The techniques used in these disciplines enable "medical detectives" both to uncover a medical problem, to evaluate the evidence about its causality or etiology, and to evaluate therapeutic interventions to combat the problem.

Descriptive epidemiology provides information on the pattern of diseases, on "who has what and how much of it," information that is essential for health care planning and rational allocation of resources. Such information may often uncover patterns of occurrence suggesting etiological relationships and can lead to preventive strategies. Such studies are usually of the cross-sectional type and lead to the formation of hypotheses which can then be tested in case-control, prospective and experimental studies. Clinical trials and other types of controlled studies serve to evaluate therapeutic modalities and other means of interventions and thus ultimately determine standards of medical practice, which in turn impact on health care planning decisions. In the following section, we will consider selected epidemiological concepts.

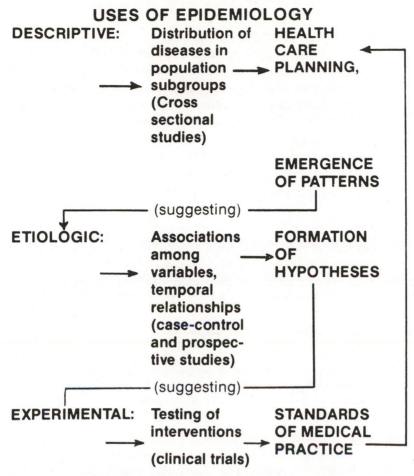

# USES OF EPIDEMIOLOGY

**DESCRIPTIVE:** Distribution of diseases in population → subgroups (Cross sectional studies) → **HEALTH CARE PLANNING,**

**EMERGENCE OF PATTERNS**

— (suggesting) —

**ETIOLOGIC:** Associations among variables, temporal relationships (case-control and prospective studies) → **FORMATION OF HYPOTHESES**

— (suggesting) —

**EXPERIMENTAL:** Testing of interventions (clinical trials) → **STANDARDS OF MEDICAL PRACTICE**

## 4.2  Some Epidemiological Concepts - Mortality Rates

In 1900, the three major causes of death were influenza or pneumonia, tuberculosis and gastroenteritis.  Today the three major causes of death are heart disease, cancer and accidents and the fourth is strokes.  Stroke deaths have decreased dramatically over the last few decades probably due to the improved control of hypertension, one of the primary risk factors for stroke.  These changing patterns of mortality reflect changing environmental conditions, a shift from acute to chronic illness, and an aging population subject to degenerative diseases.  We know this from an analysis *of rates*.

The comparison of defined *rates* among different subgroups of individuals may yield clues as to the existence of a health problem and may lead to the specification of conditions under which this identified health problem is likely to appear and flourish.

In using *rates*, the following points must be remembered:

1. A *rate* is a proportion involving a numerator and a denominator.
2. Both the numerator and the denominator must be clearly defined

In using *rates*, the following points must be remembered:

1.  A *rate* is a proportion involving a numerator and a denominator.
2.  Both the numerator and the denominator must be clearly defined so that you know to which group (denominator) your rate refers.
3.  The numerator is contained in (is a subset of) the denominator. This is in contrast to a ratio where the numerator refers to a different group from the denominator.

Mortality rates pertain to the number of deaths occurring in a particular population subgroup and often provide one of the first indications of a health problem. The following definitions are necessary before we continue our discussion:

*The Crude Annual Mortality Rate* (or death rate) is:

the *total number* of deaths during a year in the population at risk
the population at risk (usually taken as the population at mid-year)

*Cause-Specific Annual Mortality Rate* is:

number of deaths occurring due to a *particular cause* during the
          year in the population at risk
population at risk (all those alive at mid-year)

*Age-Specific Annual Mortality Rate* is:

number of deaths occurring in the given age group
          during the year in the population at risk
population at risk (those in that age group alive
                at mid-year)

A reason for taking the population at mid-year as the denominator is that a population may grow or shrink during the year in question and the mid-year population is an estimate of the average number during the year. One can however, speak of death rates over a five year period rather than a one year period and one can define the population at risk as all those alive at the beginning of the period.

## 4.3 Age-Adjusted Rates

When comparing death rates between two populations, the age composition of the populations must be taken into account. Since older people have a higher number of deaths per 1,000 people, if a population is heavily weighted by older and a comparison  between the two groups might just reflect the age discrepancy rather than an intrinsic difference in mortality experience.  One way to deal with this problem is to compare age-specific death rates, death rates specific to a particular age group.  Another way which is useful when an overall summary figure is required, is to use *age-adjusted* rates.  These are rates adjusted to what they *would be* if the two populations being compared had the same age distributions as some arbitrarily selected standard population.

For example, the table below shows the crude and age-adjusted mortality rates for the United States at four time periods.[15]  The adjustment is made to the age distribution of the population in 1940.  Thus, we see that in 1987 the age-adjusted rate was 5.4/1000, but the crude mortality rate was 8.7/1000.   This means that if in 1987 the age distribution of the population were the same as it was in 1940, then the death rate would have been only  5.4/1000 people.  The crude and age-adjusted rates for 1940 are the same because the 1940 population serves as the "standard" population whose age distribution is used as the basis for adjustment.

| Year | Crude Mortality Rate per 1,000 People | Age-Adjusted rate (to population in 1940) |
|------|---------------------------------------|-------------------------------------------|
| 1940 | 10.8 | 10.8 |
| 1960 | 9.5 | 7.6 |
| 1980 | 8.8 | 5.9 |
| 1983 | 8.6 | 5.5 |
| 1987 | 8.7 | 5.4 |

While both crude and age-adjusted rates have decreased from 1940, the decrease in the age-adjusted rate is much greater.  The percent change in crude mortality between 1940 and 1987 was (10.8-8.7)/10.8 = 19.4%, while the percent change in the age-adjusted rate was (10.8-5.4)/10.8 = 50%.  The reason for this is that the population is growing older.  For instance the proportion of persons 65 years and over doubled between 1920 and 1960, rising from 4.8% of the population in 1920 to 9.6% in 1969.

The age-adjusted rates are fictitious numbers - they do not tell you how many people actually died per 1,000, but how many *would have* died if the age compositions were the same in the two populations.  However, they are appropriate for comparison purposes.

Methods used to perform age-adjustment are described in Appendix D.

## 4.4  Incidence and Prevalence Rates

The prevalence rate and the incidence rate are two measures of morbidity (illness).

*Prevalence rate* of a disease is defined as:

$$\frac{\text{Number of persons with a disease}}{\text{Total number of persons in population at risk at a particular point in time}}$$

(This is also known as *point prevalence*, but more generally referred to just as "prevalence").

For example, the prevalence of hypertension in 1973 among black males, ages 30-69, (defined as a diastolic blood pressure of 95 mmHg or more at a blood pressure screening program conducted by the HDFP, Hypertension Detection and Follow-Up Program)[16] was calculated to be:

$$\frac{4{,}268 \text{ with DBP} > 95 \text{ mmHg}}{15{,}190 \text{ black men aged 30-69 screened}} \quad \text{X} \quad 100 \; = \; 28.1 \text{ per } 100$$

Several points are to be noted about this definition:

1.  The risk group (denominator) is clearly defined as black men, ages 30-69.
2.  The point in time is specified as time of screening.
3.  The definition of the disease is clearly specified as a diastolic blood pressure of 95 mmHg or greater. (This may include people who are treated for the disease but whose pressure is still high and those who are untreated.)
4.  The numerator is the subset of individuals in the reference group (denominator) who satisfy the definition of the disease.

The *incidence rate* is defined as:

$$\frac{\text{Number of new cases of a disease per unit of time}}{\text{Total number at risk in beginning of this time period}}$$

For example, studies have found that the ten-year incidence of a major coronary event (such as heart attack) among white men, ages 30-59, with diastolic blood pressure 105 mmHg or above at the time they were first seen, was found to be 183 per 1,000.[17] This means that among 1,000 white men, ages 30-59, who had diastolic blood pressure above 105 mmHg at the beginning of the ten-year period of observation, 183 of them had a major coronary event (heart attack or sudden death) during the next ten years. Among white men with diastolic blood pressure of <75 mmHg, the ten-year incidence of a coronary event was found to be 55/1000. Thus comparison of these two incidence rates = 183/1000 for those with high blood pressure versus 55/1000 for those with low blood pressure, may lead to the inference that elevated blood pressure is a risk factor for coronary disease.

Often one may hear the word "incidence" used when what is really meant is prevalence. You should beware of such incorrect usage. For example, you might hear or even read in a medical journal that the incidence of diabetes in 1973 was 42.6 per 1,000 individuals, ages 45-64, when what is really meant is that the prevalence was 42.6/1,000. The thing to remember is that prevalence refers to the *existence of a disease* at a specific period in time while incidence refers to *new cases* of a disease developing within a specified period of time.

Note that *mortality rate is an incidence rate* while *morbidity may be expressed as an incidence or prevalence rate*. In a chronic disease the prevalence rate is greater than the incidence rate because prevalence includes both new cases and existing cases which may have first occurred a long time ago but the afflicted patients continued to live with the condition. For a disease that is either rapidly fatal or quickly cured, incidence and prevalence may be similar. Prevalence can be established by doing a survey or a screening of a target population and counting the cases of disease existing at the time of the survey. This is a cross-sectional study.

Incidence figures are harder to obtain than prevalence figures since to ascertain incidence, one must identify a group of people free of the disease in question (known as a cohort), observe them over a period of time and determine how many develop the disease over that time period. The implementation of such a process is difficult and costly.

## 4.5 Standardized Mortality Ratio

The *standardized mortality ratio* is the ratio of the number of deaths observed to the number of deaths expected. The number expected for a particular age group for instance, is often obtained from population statistics.

$$S\ M\ R = \frac{observed\ deaths}{expected\ deaths}$$

## 4.6 Person-Years of Observation

Occasionally one sees a rate presented as some number of events *per person-years of observation*, rather than per the number of individuals observed during a specified period of time. Per-person years (or months) is useful as a unit of measurement when people are observed for different lengths of time. Suppose you are observing cohorts of people free of heart disease to determine whether the incidence of heart disease is greater for smokers than for those who quit. Quitters need to be defined, for example, as those who quit more than five years prior to the start of observation. One could define quitters differently and get different results, so it is important to specify the definition. Other considerations include controlling for the length of time smoked, (which would be a function of age at the start of smoking and age at the start of the observation period), the number of cigarettes smoked, and so forth. But for simplicity, we will assume everyone among the smokers has smoked an equal amount and everyone among the quitters has smoked an equal amount prior to quitting.

We can express the incidence rate of heart disease per some unit of time, say 10 years, as the number who developed the disease during that time, divided by the number of people we observed (number at risk). However, suppose we didn't observe everyone for the same length of time. This could occur because some people moved or died of other causes or were enrolled in the study at different times or for other reasons. In such a case we could use as our denominator the number of *person-years of observation*.

For example, if individual 1 was enrolled at time = 0 and was observed for 4 years, then lost to follow-up, he would have contributed 4 person years of observation. Ten such individuals would contribute 40 person years of observation. Another individual observed for 8 years would have contributed 8 person-years of observation and 10 such individuals would contribute 80 person-years of observation for a total of 120 person-years. If 6 cases of heart disease developed among those observed, the rate would be 6 per 120 person-years, (rather than 6/10 individuals observed). Note that if the denominator is given as person-years, you don't know if it pertains to 120 people each observed for one year, or 12 people each observed for 10 years or some combination. Another problem with this method of expressing rates is that it reflects the average experience over the time span, but it may be that the rate of heart disease is the same for smokers as for quitters within the first 3 years and the rates begin to separate after that. In any case, various statistical methods are available for use with person-year analysis. An excellent explanation of this topic is given in the book: *An Introduction to Epidemiologic Methods*, by Harold A. Kahn.

## 4.7  Sensitivity, Specificity and Related Concepts

An important way to view diagnostic and screening tests is through sensitivity analysis.

The definitions of relevant terms and symbols are:
>    T+ means positive test, T- means negative test, D+ means having disease, D- means not having disease.

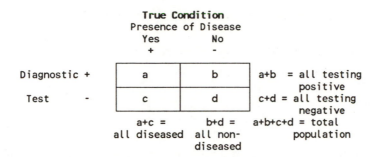

**SENSITIVITY**:  the proportion of diseased persons the test classifies as positive.

$$= \frac{a}{a+c} = P(T+ | D+); \text{ (probability of positive test, given disease)}$$

**SPECIFICITY**:  the proportion of non-diseased persons the test classifies as negative.

$$= \frac{d}{b+d} = P(T- | D-); \text{ (probability of negative test, given no disease)}$$

**FALSE-POSITIVE RATE**:  the proportion of non-diseased persons the test classifies (incorrectly) as positive.

$$= \frac{b}{b+d} = P(T+ | D-); \text{ (probability of positive test, given no disease)}$$

**FALSE-NEGATIVE RATE**:  the proportion of diseased people the test classifies (incorrectly) as negative.

$$= \frac{c}{a+c} = P(T- | D+); \text{ (probability of negative test given disease)}$$

**PREDICTIVE VALUE OF A POSITIVE TEST**:  the proportion of positive tests that identify diseased persons.

$$= \frac{a}{a+b} = P(D+ | T+); \text{ (probability of disease given positive test)}$$

**PREDICTIVE VALUE OF A NEGATIVE TEST**: the proportion of negative tests which correctly identify non-diseased people.

$$= \frac{d}{c+d} = P(D- | T-); \text{ (probability of no disease given negative test)}$$

**ACCURACY OF THE TEST**:  the proportion of all tests which are correct classifications.

$$= \frac{a+d}{a+b+c+d}$$

NOTE also the following relationships:

1.        Specificity + the false-positive rate = 1;

$$\frac{d}{b + d} \; + \; \frac{b}{b + d} = 1$$

therefore, if the specificity of a test is increased the false-positive ratio is decreased.

2.        Sensitivity + false-negative ratio = 1;

$$\frac{a}{a + c} \; + \; \frac{c}{a + c} = 1$$

therefore, if the sensitivity of a test is increased the false-negative ratio will be decreased.

*PRE-TEST PROBABILITY OF DISEASE*:  The pre-test probability of a disease is its prevalence. Knowing nothing about an individual and in the absence of a diagnostic test, the best guess of the probability that the patient has the disease, is the prevalence of the disease.

*POST-TEST PROBABILITY OF DISEASE*: *After* having the results of the test, the post-test  probability of disease if the test is normal, is c/(c+d) and if it is abnormal, the post-test probability is a/(a+b). The least is the same as the *PREDICTIVE VALUE OF A POSITIVE TEST*.

A good diagnostic test is one which improves your guess about the patient's disease status over the guess you would make based on just the general prevalence of the disease.  Of primary interest to a clinician, however, is the *predictive value of a positive test (PV+)*, which is the proportion of people who have a positive test who really have the disease:  a/(a+b), and the *predictive value of a negative test (PV-)*, which is the proportion of people with a negative test who really don't have the disease:  d/(c+d).

Sensitivity and specificity are characteristics of the test itself, but the predictive values are very much influenced by how common the disease is.  For example, for a test with 95% sensitivity and 95% specificity used to diagnose a disease which occurs only in 1% of people (or 100 out of 10,000), we would have the following:

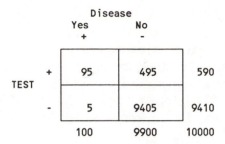

|  | Disease | | |
|---|---|---|---|
|  | Yes + | No − | |
| TEST + | 95 | 495 | 590 |
| − | 5 | 9405 | 9410 |
|  | 100 | 9900 | 10000 |

The PV+ is 95/590 = .16; that means that only 16% of all people with positive test results really have the disease; 84% do not have the disease even though the test is positive. The PV- however, is 99.9%, meaning that if a patient has a negative test result, you can be almost completely certain that he really doesn't have the disease. The practical value of a diagnostic test is dependent on a combination of sensitivity, specificity and disease prevalence, all of which determine the predictive values of test results.

If the prevalence of the disease is high, the predictive value of a positive test will also be high but a good test should have a high predictive value, even though the prevalence of the disease is low. Let us take a look at the relationship between disease prevalence and sensitivity, specificity and predictive value of a test, shown in Figure 4.2 below:

RELATIONSHIP BETWEEN DISEASE PREVALENCE, SENSITIVITY, SPECIFICITY, AND PV

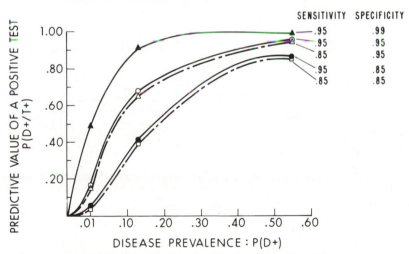

Let us for instance, consider a test that has a sensitivity of .95 and a specificity of .99. That means that this test will correctly label as diseased 95% of individuals with the disease and will correctly label as non-diseased 99% of individuals without the disease. Let us consider a disease whose prevalence is 10%, that is, 10% of the population have this disease and let us now look and see what the predictive value of a positive test is. We note that it is approximately .90 which means that 90% of individuals with a positive test will have the disease. We can see that the predictive value of a positive test, drops to approximately .70 for a test that has a sensitivity of .95 and a specificity of .95 and we can see that it further drops to approximately .40 for a test that has a sensitivity of .95 and a specificity of .85. In other words, only 40% of individuals with a positive test would truly have the disease for a test that has that particular sensitivity and specificity.

One thing you can note immediately is that *for disease of low prevalence, the predictive value of a positive test goes down rather sharply.* The other thing that you can notice almost immediately is that large difference in sensitivity makes a small difference in the predictive value of a positive test and that a small difference in specificity makes a big difference in the predictive value of a positive test. This means that the characteristic of a screening test described by specificity is more important in determining the predictive value of a positive test than is sensitivity.

Figure 4.3 below shows us a situation of a test that's virtually perfect.

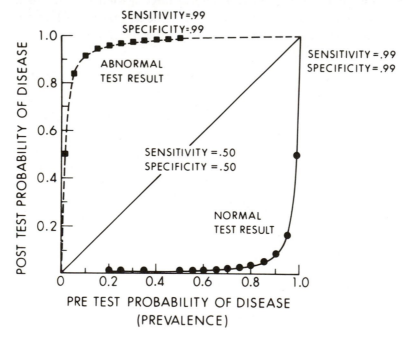

A test that has a sensitivity of .99 and a specificity of ..99 is such that at most prevalence levels of disease the probability of disease given a normal or negative test result, is very low at all prevalence of the disease. That would be a very good test and the closer we can get to that kind of situation, the better the diagnostic test is. The diagonal line in the center represents a test with a sensitivity of .50 and a specificity of .50 and that of course, is a completely useless test because you can note that at the prevalence of the disease of .4 the probability of the disease given a positive test is also .4 which is the same as the probability of the disease without doing any test, and this pertains at each prevalence level.  Therefore, such a test is completely useless while a test with sensitivity and specificity of .99 is excellent and anything in between represents different usefulness for tests.  This then, is an analytic way to look at diagnostic test procedures.

A particularly relevant example of the implications of prevalence on predictive value is the case of screening for the presence of infection with the AIDS virus.  Since this disease is invariably fatal, incurable at present, has a stigma attached to it, and entails high costs, one would not like to use a screening strategy which falsely labels people as positive for HIV, the AIDS virus.  Let us imagine that we have a test for this virus which has a sensitivity of 100% and a specificity of 99.995%, clearly a very good test.  Suppose we apply it routinely to all female blood donors, in whom the prevalence is estimated to be very low, .01%.  In comparison, suppose we also apply it to homosexual men in San Francisco in whom the prevalence is estimated to be 50%.[18]  For every 100,000 such people screened, we would have the following:

### Positive Predictive Value as a Function of Prevalence
### Test characteristics:
Sensitivity = 100%; specificity = 99.995% False positive rate = .005%

A. FEMALE BLOOD DONORS  Prevalence = .01%,
                    TRUE STATE OF NATURE
                          HIV

| | | + | - | | |
|---|---|---|---|---|---|
| SCREENING | + | 10 | 5 | 15 | PV+ = $\frac{10}{15}$ = .66667 |
| RESULT | - | 0 | 99,985 | 99,985 | |
| | | 10 | 99,990 | 100,000 | |

B. MALE HOMOSEXUALS                    Prevalence = 50%,
                    TRUE STATE OF NATURE
                          HIV

| | | + | - | | |
|---|---|---|---|---|---|
| SCREENING | + | 50,000 | 3 | 50,003 | PV+ = $\frac{50,000}{50,003}$ = .99994 |
| RESULT | - | 0 | 49,997 | 49,997 | |
| | | 50,000 | 50,000 | 100,000 | |

While in both groups all those who really had the disease would be identified, among female blood donors, one third of all people who tested positive would really not have the disease; among male homosexuals only 6 out of 10,000 people with a positive test would be falsely labeled.

## 4.8  Cut-Off Point and Its Effects on Sensitivity and Specificity

We have been discussing sensitivity and specificity as characteristic of a
diagnostic test; however, they can be modified by the choice of the *cut-off point
between normal and abnormal*.  For example, we may want to diagnose patients
as hypertensive or normotensive by their diastolic blood pressure.  Let us say
that anyone with a diastolic pressure of 90 mmHg. or more will be classified as
"hypertensive".  Since blood pressure is a continuous and variable characteristic,
on any one measurement, a usually non-hypertensive individual may have a
diastolic blood pressure of 90 mmHg. or more and similarly, a truly hypertensive
individual may have a single measure less than 90 mmHg. with a cut-off point
of 90 mmHg.  We will call some non-hypertensive individuals as hypertensive
and these will be false-positive.  We will also label some hypertensive individuals
as normotensive and these will be false-negatives.  If we had a more stringent
cut-off point, say, 105 mmHg., we would call fewer non-hypertensives as
hypertensive since fewer normotensive individuals would have such a high
reading, (and have fewer false-positive).  However, we would have more
false-negatives (i.e., more of our truly hypertensive people might register as
having diastolic blood pressure less than 105 mmHg. on any single occasion).
These concepts are illustrated in Figure 4.4.

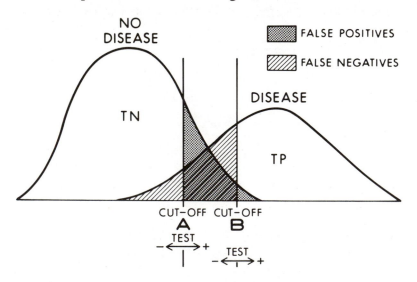

CUTOFF  A :  GREATER SENSITIVITY; LOWER SPECIFICITY; MORE
                    FALSE POSITIVES.

CUTOFF  B :  LOWER SENSITIVITY; HIGHER SPECIFICITY; MORE
                    FALSE NEGATIVES

There are two population distributions: the diseased and non-diseased, and they overlap on the measure of interest, whether it is blood pressure, blood glucose, or other laboratory values. There are very few screening tests which have no overlap between normal and diseased individuals.

One objective in deciding on a cut-off point, is to strike the proper balance between false-positive and false-negatives. As you can see in the figure, when the cut-off point is at A, all values to the right of A are called positive (patient is considered to have the disease). In fact, however, the patient with a value at the right of cut-off A could come from the population of non-diseased people, since a proportion of people who are perfectly normal, may still have values higher than those above A, as seen in the normal curve. The area to the right of A under the no disease curve represents the false positive.

If an individual has a test value to the left of cut-off A, he may be a true negative or he may be a false-negative because a proportion of individuals with the disease can still have values lower than cut-off A. The area under the "disease" curve to the left of cut-off A represents the proportion of false-negatives.

If we move the cut-off point from A to B, we see that we decrease the area to the right of the cut-off, thereby decreasing the number of false-positive, but increasing the number of false negatives. Correspondingly, with cut-off A, we have a greater probability of identifying the truly diseased correctly, i.e., pick up more true positive, thereby giving the test with cut-off A greater sensitivity. With cut-off B, we are less likely to pick up the true positive (lower sensitivity) but more likely to correctly identify the true negatives (higher specificity).

Thus, by shifting the cut-off point beyond which we call a test positive, we can change the sensitivity and specificity characteristics of the test. The choice of cut-off, unless there is some special physiological reason may be based on consideration of the relative consequences of having too many false-positive or too many false-negatives. In a screening test for cancer, for example, it would be desirable to have a test of high sensitivity (and few false-negatives), since failure to detect this condition early is often fatal. In a mass screening test for a less serious condition or for one where early detection is not critical, it may be more desirable to have a high specificity in order not to overburden the health care delivery system with too many false-positive. Cost consideration may also enter into the choice of cut-off point.

The relationship between sensitivity (the ability to correctly identify the diseased individuals) and the false-positive fractions, is shown in Figure 4.5.

This is called the Receiver Operating Characteristic Curve of the test (ROC Curve). Often we can select the cut-off point between normal and abnormal depending on the trade off we are willing to make between sensitivity and the proportion of false-positive.

We can see that with cut-off A, while we can detect a greater percentage of truly diseased individuals, we will also have, a greater proportion of false-positive results, while with cut-off B, we will have fewer false-positive but will be less likely to detect the truly diseased. Screening tests should have corresponding ROC Curves drawn.

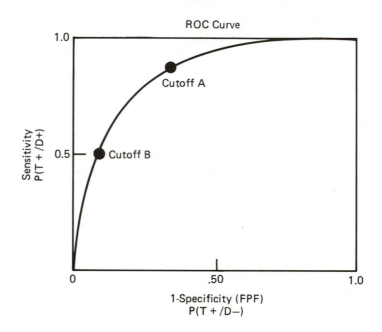

## 4.9  Dependent, Independent and Confounding Variables

In research studies we want to quantify the relationship between one set of variables which we may think of as predictors or determinants and some outcome or criterion variable in which we are interested. This outcome variable, which it is our objective to explain, is the dependent variable.

A *dependent variable* is a factor whose value depends on the level of another factor which is termed an *independent variable*. In the example of cigarette smoking and lung cancer mortality, duration and/or number of cigarettes smoked are independent variables upon which the lung cancer mortality depends (thus, lung cancer mortality is the dependent variable).

A *confounding variable* is one which is closely associated with both the independent variable and the outcome of interest. For example, a confounding variable in studies of coffee and heart disease may be smoking. Since coffee drinkers are also often smokers, if a study found a relationship between coffee drinking (the independent variable) and development of heart disease, (the dependent variable), it could really mean that it is the smoking that causes heart disease, rather than the coffee. In this example, smoking is the confounding variable.

If *both* the confounding variable and the independent variable are closely associated with the dependent variable, then the observed relationship between the independent and dependent variables may really be a reflection of the *true* relationship between the confounding variable and the dependent variable. An intuitive way to look at this is to imagine that if a confounding variable were perfectly associated with an independent variable, it could be substituted for it. It is important to account or adjust for confounding variables *in the design and statistical analysis of studies* in order to avoid wrong inferences. Various approaches to dealing with potential confounders are discussed in the more advanced texts listed at the end.

## 4.10  Matching

One approach to dealing with potential confounders is to match subjects in the two groups on the confounding variable. In the example discussed above concerning studies of coffee and heart disease, we might match subjects on their smoking history, since smoking may be a confounder of the relationship between coffee and heart disease. Whenever we enrolled a coffee-drinker into the study, we would determine if that person was a smoker. If the patient was a smoker, the next patient who would be enrolled who was not a coffee drinker (i.e. a member of the comparison group), would also have to be a smoker. For each coffee-drinking non-smoker, a non-coffee-drinking non-smoker would be enrolled. In this way we would have the same number of smokers in the two groups. This is known as *one-to-one matching*. There are other ways to match and these are discussed more fully in the references given in back, especially in *Statistical Methods for Comparative Studies* by Anderson et al.John Wiley & Sons, 1980, and in *Causal Relationships in Medicine* by J. Mark Elwood, Oxford University Press, 1988.

In case-control studies finding an appropriate comparison group may be difficult. For example, suppose an investigator is studying the effect of coffee on pancreatic cancer. The investigator chooses as control patients in the hospital at the same time and in the same ward as the cases, but with a diagnosis other than cancer. It is possible that patients hospitalized for gastrointestinal problems other than cancer might have voluntarily given up coffee drinking because it bothered their stomachs. In such a situation, the coffee drinking habits of the two groups might be similar and the investigator might not find a greater association of coffee drinking with cases than with controls. A more appropriate group might be patients in a different ward, say an orthopedic ward. But, here one would have to be careful to match on age, since orthopedic patients may be younger than cases - if the hospital happens to be in a ski area for example where reckless skiing leads to broken legs, or they may be substantially older than the cases if there are many patients with hip replacements due to falls in the elderly.

It needs to be pointed out that the factor which is matched cannot be evaluated in terms of its relationship to outcome. Thus, if we are comparing two groups of women for the effect of vitamin A intake on cervical cancer and we do a case-control study in which we enroll cases of cervical cancer and controls matched on age we will not be able to say from this study whether age is related to cervical cancer. This is because we have ensured that the age distributions are the same in both the case and control groups by matching on age, so obviously, we will not be able to find differences in age between the groups.

Some statisticians believe that matching is often done unnecessarily and that if you have a large enough study, simple randomization, or stratified randomization, is adequate to ensure a balanced distribution of confounding factors. A good discussion of matching can be found in the book *Methods in Observational Epidemiology*, by Kelsey, Thompson and Evans.

## 4.11  Measures of Relative Risk - Relative Risk and the Framingham Study

In epidemiological studies we are often interested in knowing how much more likely an individual is to develop a disease if he or she is exposed to a particular factor than the individual who is not so exposed. A simple measure of such likelihood is called *Relative Risk (RR)*. It is the ratio of two incidence rates: *the rate of development of the disease for people with the factor, divided by the rate of development of the disease for people without the factor*. Suppose we wish to determine the effect of high blood pressure (hypertension) on the development of cardiovascular disease (CVD). To obtain the relative risk we need to calculate the incidence rates. We can use the data from a classic prospective study, the *Framingham Heart Study*.[19]

This was a pioneering prospective epidemiological study of a population sample in the small town of Framingham, Massachusetts. Beginning in 1948 a *cohort* of people was selected to be followed up biennially. The term cohort refers to a group of individuals followed longitudinally over a period of time. A birth cohort, for example, would be the population of individuals born in a given year. The Framingham cohort was a sample of people chosen at the beginning of the study period, and included men and women aged 30 to 62 years at the start of the study. These individuals were observed over a 20 year period, and morbidity and mortality associated with cardiovascular disease were determined. A standardized hospital record and death certificate were obtained, clinic examination was repeated at two-year intervals and the major concern of the Framingham Study has been to evaluate the relationship of characteristics determined in *well* persons to the subsequent development of disease.

Through this study "risk factors" for cardiovascular disease were identified. The *risk factors* are antecedent physiological characteristics or dietary and living habits, whose presence increases the individual's probability of developing cardiovascular disease at some future time. Among the most important predictive factors identified in the Framingham Study were *elevated blood pressure, elevated serum cholesterol, and cigarette smoking*. Elevated blood glucose and abnormal resting electrocardiogram findings are also predictive of future cardiovascular disease.

*Relative risk* can be determined by the following calculation:

incidence rate of cardiovascular disease (new cases) over a specified period of time among people free of CVD at beginning of the study period *who have* the risk factor in question (e.g., high blood pressure)

---

incidence rate of CVD in the given time period among people free of CVD initially, who *do not have* the risk factor in question (normal blood pressure)

From the Framingham data we calculate for men in the study the

RR of CVD = <u>353.2/10,000 persons at risk with definite hypertension</u> =
within 18             123.9/10,000 persons at risk with no hypertension
years after
first examination

$$\frac{353.2}{123.9} = 2.85$$

This means that a man with definite hypertension is 2.85 time more likely to develop CVD in an 18 year period than a man who does not have hypertension. For women the Relative Risk is

$$\frac{187.9}{57.3} = 3.28$$

This means that hypertension carries a somewhat greater relative risk for women. But note that the *absolute* risk for persons with definite hypertension (i.e. the incidence of CVD) is greater for men than for women, being 353.2 per 10,000 men versus 187.9 per 10,000 women.

The incidence rates given above have been age-adjusted. Age adjustment is discussed in Section 4.3. Often one may want to adjust for other variables such as smoking status, diabetes, cholesterol levels and other factors which may also be related to outcome. This may be accomplished by multiple logistic regression analysis which are discussed fully in the more advanced texts listed in the references section, and described here in Section 4.13.

## 4.12 Calculation of Relative Risk From Prospective Studies

Relative risk can be determined directly from prospective studies by constructing a 2x2 table as follows[20]:

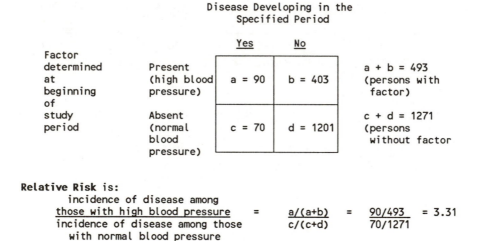

**Relative Risk is:**

$$\frac{\text{incidence of disease among those with high blood pressure}}{\text{incidence of disease among those with normal blood pressure}} = \frac{a/(a+b)}{c/(c+d)} = \frac{90/493}{70/1271} = 3.31$$

## 4.13 Odds Ratio:  Estimate of Relative Risk From Case-Control Studies

A case-control study is one in which the investigator seeks to establish an association between the presence of a characteristic (a risk factor) and the occurrence of a disease, *by starting out with a sample of diseased persons and a control group of non-diseased persons and by noting the presence or absence of the characteristic in each of these two groups.* It can be illustrated by constructing a 2x2 table as follows:

Disease

|              |         | Present | Absent |
|--------------|---------|---------|--------|
| Risk Factor  | Present |    a    |   b    |
|              | Absent  |    c    |   d    |

a + c
number of
persons with
disease

b + d
number of persons
without disease

The objective is to determine if the proportion of persons with the disease who have the factor is greater than the proportion of persons without the disease who have the factor. In other words, it is desired to know whether $a/(a + c)$ is greater than $b/(b + d)$.

*Case-control studies* are often referred to as *retrospective studies* because the investigator must gather data on the *independent* variables retrospectively. The dependent variable - the presence of disease - is obtained at time of sampling. In prospective studies the independent variables are measured at time of sampling and the dependent variable is measured at some future time (i.e. when the disease develops). The real distinction between case-control or retrospective studies and prospective studies has to do with selecting individuals for the study - those with and without the disease in case-control/retrospective studies, and those with and without the factor of interest in prospective studies.

Since in prospective studies *we sample the people with the characteristic of interest and the people without the characteristic*, we can obtain the relative risk *directly* by calculating the incidence rates of disease in these two groups. In case-control studies, however, *we sample patients with and without the disease*, and note the presence or absence of the characteristic of interest in these two groups; we do not have a direct measure of *incidence* of disease. Nevertheless, making certain assumptions, we can make some approximations to what the relative risk would be if we could measure incidence rates through a prospective study. These approximations hold best for diseases of *low incidence*.

To estimate relative risk from case-control studies note that:

$$\frac{\dfrac{a}{a + b}}{\dfrac{c}{c + d}} = \frac{a(c + d)}{c(a + b)}$$

Now assume that since the disease is not all that common, c is small in relation to d (in other words among people without the risk factor there aren't all that many who will get the disease, relative to the number of people who will not get it). Assume also that a is small relative to b since even among people with the risk factor, not all that many will get the disease in comparison to the number who won't get it). In fact, assume that these are negligible. Then the terms in the parentheses become d in the numerator and b in the denominator so that:

$$\frac{a(c+d)}{c(a+b)} \, reduces \, to: \qquad OR = \frac{ad}{bc}$$

This is known as the *odds ratio* and is a good estimate of relative risk when the disease is rare.

An example of how the odds ratio is calculated is shown below. In a case-control study of lung cancer the table below was obtained[21]:

|  | Patients With Lung Cancer | Matched Controls With Other Diseases |
|---|---|---|
| Smokers of 14-24 cigarettes daily | 475     a | 431     b |
| Non-smokers | 7     c | 61     d |
|  | (persons with disease) | (persons without disease) |

The odds ratio, as an estimate of the relative risk of developing lung cancer for people who smoke 15-24 cigarettes a day, compared to non-smokers is:

$$Odds \, ratio = \frac{475 \times 61}{431 \times 7} = 9.60 = estimate \, of \, relative \, risk$$

This means that smokers of 15-24 cigarettes daily are 9.6 times more likely to get lung cancer than are non-smokers.

We can also put confidence limits on the odds ratio, shown in Appendix E.

### 4.14 Multiple Logistic Regression

Multiple logistic regression analysis is used to calculate the probability of an event happening as a function of several independent variables. The equation takes the form of:

$$P(event) = \frac{1}{1+e^{-k}} \quad where \; k = C_0 + C_1 X_1 + C_2 X_2 + C_3 X_3 .... C_m X_m$$

Each $X_i$ is a particular independent variable and the corresponding coefficients, C's, are calculated from the data obtained in the study. For example, let us take the Framingham data for the probability of a man developing cardiovascular disease within 8 years. Cardiovascular disease (CVD) was defined as coronary heart disease brain infarction, intermittent claudication or congestive heart failure.

$$P(CVD) = \frac{1}{1 + e^{-[-19.77 + .37(age) - .002(age)^2 + .026(chol) + .016(SBP) + .558(smoking) + 1.053(LVH) + .602(Gli) - .0003}}$$

chol = serum cholesterol

SBP = systolic blood pressure

smoking = 1 if yes, 0 if no

LVH = left ventricular hypertrophy, 1 if yes, 0 if no

Gli = Glucose intolerance, 1 if yes, 0 if no

For example, suppose we consider a 50 year old male whose cholesterol is 200, systolic blood pressure is 160, who smokes, has no LVH and no glucose intolerance. When we multiply the coefficients by this individual's values on the independent variables and do the necessary calculations we come up with a probability of .17. this means that this individual has 17 chances in a 100 of developing some form of cardiovascular disease within the next 8 years.

The coefficients from a multiple logistic regression analysis can be used to calculate the odds ratio for one factor while controlling for all the other factors. The way to do this is to take the natural log e raised to the coefficient for the variable of interest, if the variable is a dichotomous one (i.e. coded as 1 or 0). For example, the odds of cardiovascular disease for smokers relative to non-smokers among males, while controlling for age, cholesterol, systolic blood pressure, left ventricular hypertrophy and glucose intolerance is $e^{.558} = 1.75$. This means that a person who smokes has 1.75 times higher risk of getting CVD than the one who doesn't smoke if these two individuals are equal with respect to the other variables in the equation. This is equivalent to saying that the smoker's risk is 75% higher than the non-smoker's. If we want compare the odds of someone with a systolic blood pressure of 200 vs. someone with systolic blood pressure of 120, all other factors being equal, we calculate it as follows:

$$O.R. = e^{\beta(200-120)} = e^{.016(80)} = e^{1.28} = 3.6$$

The man with systolic blood pressure of 200 is 3.6 times more likely to develop disease than the one with pressure of 120.

Multiple logistic regression analysis has become widely used largely due to the advent of high speed computers, since calculating the coefficients requires a great deal of computer power. Statistical packages are available which will now do this on personal computers.

## 4.15  Cross-Sectional Versus Longitudinal Looks at Data

Prospective studies are sometimes also known as longitudinal studies, since people are followed longitudinally, over time. Examination of longitudinal data may lead to quite different inferences than those to be obtained from cross-sectional looks at data. For example, consider age and blood pressure.

Cross-sectional studies have repeatedly shown that the average systolic blood pressure is higher in each successive ten-year age group while diastolic pressure increases for age groups up to age 50 and then reaches a plateau. One cannot, from these types of studies, say that blood pressure rises with age because the pressures measured for 30 year old men for example, were not obtained on the same individuals ten years later when they were 40, but were obtained for a different set of 40 year olds. To determine the effect of age on blood pressure we would need to take a longitudinal or prospective look at the same individuals as they get older. One interpretation of the curve observed for diastolic blood pressure, for instance, might be that individuals over 60 who had very high diastolic pressures died off, leaving only those individuals with lower pressure alive long enough to be included in the sample of those having their blood pressure measured in the cross-sectional look.

The following diagrams (Figure 4.6) illustrate the possible impact of a "cohort effect", a cross-sectional view and a longitudinal view of the same data. (Letters indicate groups of individuals examined in a particular year).

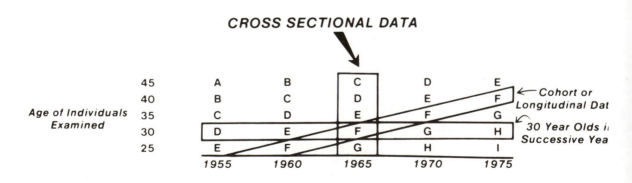

Year of Examination

If you take the blood pressure of all groups in 1965, and compare group F to group D, you will have a cross-sectional comparison of 30 year olds with 40 year olds at a given point in time. If you compare group F in 1965 with group F (same individuals) in 1975, you will have a longitudinal comparison. If you compare group F in 1965 with group H in 1975, you will have a comparison of blood pressures of 30 year olds at different points in time (a horizontal look).

These comparisons can lead to quite different conclusions, as is shown by the following schematic examples (Figure 4.7) using fictitious numbers to represent average diastolic blood pressure.

Figure 4.7

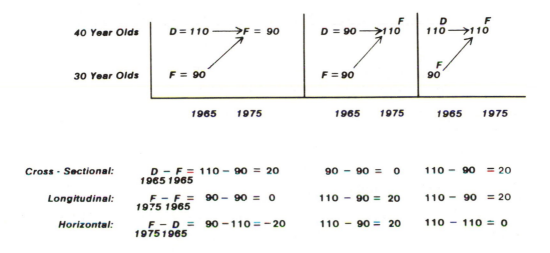

In example (1) measurements in 1965 indicate that average diastolic blood pressure for 30 year olds (group F) was 90 mmHg and for 40 year olds (group D), it was 110 mmHg. Looking at group F ten years later, when they were 40 years old, indicates their mean diastolic blood pressure was 90 mmHg. The following calculations result:

cross-sectional look:  $D_{1965} - F_{1965} = 110 - 90 = 20$

   conclusion: 40 year olds have higher blood pressure than 30 year olds (by 20 mmHg).

*longitudinal look*:          F     -     F          =  90-90= 0
                             1975        1965

**conclusion**: Blood pressure does not rise with age

*horizontal look*:            F     -     D          =  90-110= -20
(cohort comparisons)        1975        1965

**conclusion**: 40 year olds in 1975 have lower blood pressure than 40 year olds did in 1965

*A possible interpretation*:  Blood pressure does not rise with age, but different environmental forces were operating for the F cohort, than for the D cohort. In example (2) we have:

*cross-sectional look*:   D      -     F          = 90-90= 0  mmHg
                        1965         1965

**conclusion**: from cross-sectional data, we conclude that blood pressure is not higher with older age.

*longitudinal look*:          F     -     F          = 110-90=20
                             1975        1965

**conclusion**: from longitudinal data we conclude that blood pressure goes up with age

*horizontal look*:            F     -     D          = 110-90= 20
                             1975        1965

**conclusion**: 40 year olds in 1975 have higher blood pressure than 40 year olds in 1965

*A possible interpretation*:  Blood pressure does rise with age and different environmental factors operated on the F cohort than on the D cohort.

In example (3) we have:

*cross-sectional look*:   D      -     F          =110-90= 20
                        1965         1965

**conclusion**: cross-sectionally, there was an increase in blood pressure for 40 year olds over that for 30 year olds.

*longitudinal look*:          F      -      F      = 110-90=20
                           1975         1965

   **conclusion**: longitudinally it is seen that blood
   pressure increases with increasing age

*horizontal look*:           F      -      D      = 110-110= 0
                           1975         1965

   **conclusion**: there was no change in blood pressure
   among 40 year olds over the ten year period.

*A possible interpretation*:  Blood pressure does go up with age (supported by both
longitudinal and cross-sectional data) and environmental factors affect both
cohorts similarly.

# Section 5

## MOSTLY ABOUT CLINICAL TRIALS

*"It is no easy task to pitch one's way from truth to truth through besetting errors."*

Peter Marc Latham, 1789-1875

*A randomized clinical trial is a prospective experiment*, to compare two or more interventions against a control group in order to determine the effectiveness of the interventions. A clinical trial may compare the value of a drug versus a placebo. A placebo is an inert substance that looks like the drug being tested. It may compare a new therapy versus a currently standard therapy. It may compare surgical versus medical intervention. It may also compare two methods of teaching reading, two methods of psychotherapy. The principles apply to any situation in which the issue of who is exposed to which condition is under the control of the experimenter and the method of assignment is through randomization.

### 5.1 Features of Randomized Clinical Trials

1.  There is a group of patients who are designated study patients. All criteria must be set forth and met before a potential candidate can be considered eligible for the study. Any exclusions must be specified.

2.  Any reasons for excluding a potential patient from participating in the trial must be specified prior to starting the study. Otherwise, unintentional bias may enter. For example, supposing you are comparing coronary bypass surgery with the use of a new drug for the treatment of coronary artery disease. Suppose a patient comes along who is eligible for the study and gets assigned to the surgical treatment. Suppose you now discover the patient has kidney disease. You decide to exclude him from the study because you think he may not survive the surgery with damaged kidneys. If you end up systematically excluding all the sicker patients from the surgical treatment, you

may bias the results in favor of the healthier patients who have a better chance of survival in any case. In this example, kidney disease should be an *exclusion criterion applied to the patients before they are assigned to any treatment group.*

3.  Once a patient is eligible he or she is randomly assigned to the experimental or control group. Random assignment is not "haphazard" assignment but rather it means that each person has an equal chance of being an experimental or control patient. It is usually accomplished by the use of a table of random numbers, described later.

4.  Clinical trials often compare a drug or treatment with placebo, i.e., with the administration of a pill or a treatment under exactly the same conditions as the administration of the therapeutic agent under study, but not containing the therapeutic agent (it may contain sugar, or some inert substance). However, clinical trials may also compare two treatments with each other.

5.  The group that receives the placebo (no treatment group) is the control group against which comparisons will be made. It is essential that the control group be as similar to the treatment group as possible so that differences in outcome can be attributed to differences in treatment and not to different characteristics of the two groups. Randomization helps to achieve this comparability.

6.  Clinical trials may be double-blind, in which neither the treating physician nor the patient knows whether the patient is getting the experimental treatment or the placebo; they may be single-blind, in which the treating physician knows which group the patient is in but the patient does not know. A double-blind study contains the least bias but sometimes is not possible to do for ethical or practical reasons. For example, the doctor may need to know the group to which the patient belongs so that medication may be adjusted for the welfare of the patient. There are also trials in which both patients and physicians know the treatment group, as in trials comparing radical mastectomy versus lumpectomy for treatment of breast cancer. When mortality is the outcome the possible bias introduced is minimal.

## 5.2  Purposes of Randomization

The basic principle in designing clinical trials or any scientific investigation is to *avoid systematic bias*.  When it is not known which variables may affect the outcome of an experiment, the best way to avoid systematic bias is to assign individuals into groups randomly.  *Randomization* is intended to insure an approximately equal distribution of variables, among the various groups of individuals being studied.  For instance, if you are studying the effect of an anti-diabetic drug and you know that cardiac risk factors affect mortality among diabetics, you would not want all the patients in the control group to have heart disease, since that would clearly bias the results.  By assigning patients randomly to the drug and the control group, you can expect that the distribution of patients with cardiac problems will be comparable in the two groups.  Since there are many variables which are unknown, but which may have a bearing on the results, randomization is insurance against unknown and unintentional bias.  Of course, when dealing with variables known to be relevant, one can take these into account by *stratifying and then randomizing within the strata*.  For instance, age is a variable relevant to diabetes outcome.  To stratify by age, you might select four age groups for your study:  35-44, 45-54, 55-64, 65 plus.  Each group is considered a stratum.  When a patient enters into the clinical trial his age stratum is first determined and then he is randomly assigned to either experimental or control groups.  Sex is another variable that is often handled by stratification.

Another purpose of randomization has to do with the fact that the statistical techniques used to compare results among the groups of patients under study are valid under certain assumptions arising out of randomization.  The mathematical reasons for this can be found in the more advanced texts listed in the recommended readings.

It should be remembered that sometimes randomization fails to result in comparable groups due to chance.  This can present a major problem in the interpretation of results, since differences in outcome may reflect differences in the composition of the groups on baseline characteristics rather than the effect of intervention.  Statistical methods are available for adjustment for baseline characteristics which are known to be related to outcome. Some of these methods, discussed extensively in the texts listed at the end of this book, are: logistic regression, Cox proportional hazards model, multiple regression analyses.

## 5.3  How to Perform Randomized Assignment

Random assignment into an experimental group or a control group means that each eligible individual has an equal chance of being in each of the two groups. This is often accomplished by the use of random number tables.  For example, an excerpt from such a table is shown below:

| 48461 | 70436 | 04282 |
|-------|-------|-------|
| 76537 | 59584 | 69173 |

Its use might be as follows. All even-numbered persons are assigned to the treatment group and all odd-numbered persons are assigned to the control groups. The first person to enter the study is given the first number in the list, the next person gets the next number and so on. Thus, the first person is given number 48461, which is an odd number and assigns the patient to the control group. The next person is given 76537; this is also an odd number so he too belongs to the control group. The next three people to enter the study all have even numbers and they are in the experimental group. In the long run, there will be an equal number of patients in each of the two groups.

## 5.4  Two-Tail Tests Versus One-Tail Test

A clinical trial is designed to test a particular hypothesis. One often sees the phrase in research articles: "Significant at the .05 level, two tail test". Recall that in a previous section we discussed the concept of the "null hypothesis" which states that there is no difference between two groups on a measure of interest. We said that in order to test this hypothesis we would gather data so that we could decide whether we should reject the hypothesis of no difference in favor of some alternate hypothesis. *A two-tail test versus a one-tail test refers to the alternate hypothesis* posed. For example, suppose you are interested in comparing the mean cholesterol level of a group treated with a cholesterol lowering drug to the mean of a control group given a placebo. You would collect the appropriate data from a well designed study and you would set up the null hypothesis as:

$H_0$:mean cholesterol in treated group = mean cholesterol control group.
　　　　　You may choose as the alternate hypothesis:
$H_A$:mean cholesterol in treated group is *greater than* the mean in controls.

Under this circumstance, you would reject the null hypothesis in favor of the alternate hypothesis if the observed mean for women were sufficiently *greater* than the observed mean for men to lead you to the conclusion that such a great difference in that direction is not likely to have occurred by chance alone. This then would then be a one-tail test of the null hypothesis.

If however, your alternate hypothesis were that the mean cholesterol level for females is *different* from the mean cholesterol level for males, then you would reject the null hypothesis in favor of the alternate, *either* if the mean for women *were sufficiently greater* than the mean for men *or* if the mean for women *were sufficiently lower* than the mean for men. The direction of the difference is not specified. In medical research it is more common to use a two-tail test of significance since we often do not know in which direction a difference may turn out to be even though we may think we know before we start the experiment. In any case, it is important to report whether we are using a one-tail or a two-tail test.

## 5.5 Regression Toward the Mean

When you select from a population those individuals who have high blood pressure and then at a later time measure their blood pressure again, the average of the second measurements will tend to be lower than the average of the first measurements and will be closer to the mean of the original population from which these individuals were drawn. If between the first and second measurements you have instituted some treatment, you may incorrectly attribute the decline of average blood pressure in the group to the effects of treatment, whereas part of that decline  may be due to the phenomenon called *regression toward the mean*. (That is one reason why a placebo control group is most important for comparison of effects of treatment above and beyond that caused by regression to the mean.)  Regression to the mean occurs when you select out a group because individuals have values which fall above some criterion level, as in screening. It is due to variability of measurement error. Consider blood pressure.

The observed value of blood pressure is the person's true value plus some unknown amount of error. The assumption is that people's measured blood pressure is normally distributed around the mean of their true but unknown value of blood pressure. Suppose we will only take people into our study if their blood pressure is 160 or more. Now suppose someone's true systolic blood pressure is 150, but we measure it 160. We select that person for our study group just because his measured value is high. However, the next time we measure his blood pressure, he is likely to be closer to his true value of 150 than the first time. (If he had been close to his true value of 150 the first time, we would never have selected him for our study to begin with, since he would have been below our cut point. So he must have had a large error at that first measurement). Since these errors are normally distributed around his true mean of 150, the next time, we are more likely to get a lower error and thus a lower measured blood pressure than the 160 which caused us to select him.

Suppose now that we select an entire subgroup of people who have high values. The averages of the second measurements of these selected people will tend to be lower than the average of their first measurements, and closer to the average of the entire group from which we selected them. The point is that people who have the highest values the first time, do not always have the highest values the second time because the correlation between the first and second measurement is not perfect. Similarly, if we select out a group of people because of low values on some characteristic, the average of the second measurements on these people will be higher than the average of their first measurements, and again closer to the mean of the whole group.

Another explanation of this phenomenon may be illustrated by the following example of tossing a die. Imagine that you toss a die 360 times. Whenever the die lands on a five or a six, you will toss the die again. We are interested in three different averages: 1) the mean of the first 360 tosses; 2) the mean of the tosses which will result in our tossing again; and 3) the mean of the second tosses. Our results are shown on the opposite page.

From the first toss we only pick the two highest numbers and their mean is 5.5. There will be 120 times when the die landed on 5 or 6 which causes us to toss again, but on the 2nd toss the result can freely vary between 1 and 6. Therefore, the mean of the 2nd toss must be lower than the mean of the group we selected from the first toss just because it had the high values.

| 1st toss | | 2nd toss | |
|---|---|---|---|
| result | # of times result is obtained | result | # of times result is obtained |
| 1 | 60 | | |
| 2 | 60 | | |
| 3 | 60 | | |
| 4 | 60 | | |
| | | 1 | 20 |
| 5 | **60** | 2 | 20 |
| 6 | **60** | 3 | 20 |
| | | 4 | 20 |
| | | 5 | 20 |
| | | 6 | 20 |

Mean of 360 tosses = 3.5    Mean of the 2nd toss = 5.5

Mean of the tosses
which landed 5 or 6 = 5.5

## 5.6 Survival Analysis - Life Table Methods

Survival analysis of data should be used when the follow-up times differ widely for different people or when they enter the study at different times. It can get rather complex and the following section is intended only to introduce the concepts. Suppose you want to compare the survival of patients treated by two different methods and suppose you have the data shown below.[23] We will analyze it by using the Kaplan-Meier survival curves.

## DEATHS AT A GIVEN MONTH IN:

### Group A : 4, 5+, 9, 11, 13     Group B: 2, 3, 4, 5, 6+

(The + means that the patient was lost to follow-up and last seen alive at that month.)
In each group 4 patients had died by one year, and one was seen alive some time during that year, so we don't know whether that patient was dead or alive at the end of the year. If we looked at the data in this way, we would have to say that the survival by one year was the same in both groups.

|  | Group A | Group B |
|---|---|---|
| Dead | 4 | 4 |
| Alive | 1 | 1 |
| Survival Rate | 20% | 20% |

However, a more appropriate way to analyze such data is through *survival curves*. The points for the curves are calculated as shown in the table below.

GROUP A

| Case # | Pt ID | Time Mos | Status | # Pts. Enter | Prop Dead ($q_i$ = =dead =entered) | Prop Surv. ($P_1$ = $1-q_i$) | Cum Surv. $P_i$ = $P_{i-1} \times P_i$ |
|---|---|---|---|---|---|---|---|
| 1 | 1 | 4 | dead | 5 | 1/5=0.2 | 0.8 | 1x.8=.8 |
| 2 | 2 | 5 | surv | 4 | 0/4=0.0 | 1 | .8x1=.8 |
| 3 | 3 | 9 | dead | 3 | 1/3=0.33 | 0.67 | .8x.67=.53 |
| 4 | 4 | 11 | dead | 2 | 1/2=0.5 | 0.5 | .53x.5=.27 |
| 5 | 5 | 13 | dead | 1 | 1/1=1.0 | 0 | .27x0=0 |

GROUP B

| Case # | Pt ID | Time Mos | Status | # Pts. Enter | Prop Dead | Prop Surv. | Cum Surv. |
|---|---|---|---|---|---|---|---|
| 1 | 1 | 2 | dead | 5 | 1/5=0.2 | 0.8 | 1x.8=.8 |
| 2 | 2 | 3 | dead | 4 | 1/4=0.25 | 0.75 | .8x.75=.6 |
| 3 | 3 | 4 | dead | 3 | 1/3=0.33 | 0.67 | .6x.67=.4 |
| 4 | 4 | 5 | dead | 2 | 1/2=0.5 | 0.5 | .4x.5=.2 |
| 5 | 5 | 6 | surv | 1 | 0/1=0.0 | 1 | .2x.1=.2 |

First of all, the patients are placed in order of the time of their death or the last time they were seen alive. Let us go through the third row as an example. The third patient died at 9 months (columns 2 and 3). At the beginning of the 9th months there were 3 patients at risk of dying (out of the total of 5 patients who entered the study). This is because one of the 5 patients had already died in the 4th month (case #1), and one was last seen alive at the 5th month (case # 2), and so wasn't available to be observed. Out of these 3 patients at risk in the beginning of the 9th month, 1 died (case # 3). So the probability of dying in the 9th months is 1/3 and we call this $q_i$ where i in this case refers to the 9th month. Therefore the proportion surviving in the 9th month is $p_i = 1 - q_i = 1 - .33 = .67$. The cumulative proportion surviving means the proportion surviving up through the 9th month. To survive through the 9th month, a patient had to have survived to the end of month 8 *and* have survived in month 9. Thus, it is equal to the cumulative probability of surviving *up to* the 9th month, (which is .8, from column 7 row 2) *and* surviving in the 9th month, (which is .67). We multiply these probabilities to get .8 x .67 = .53 as the probability of surviving through the 9th month. If we plot these points as in Figure 5.1, we note that the two survival curves look quite different and that group A did a lot better.

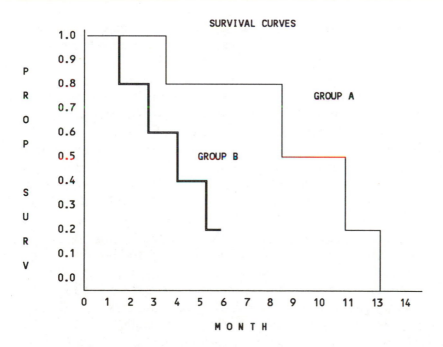

Survival analysis gets more complicated when we assume that patients who have been lost to follow-up in a given interval of time would have died at the same rate as those patient on whom we had information. Alternatively, we can make the calculations by assuming they all died within the interval in which they were lost to follow-up, or they all survived during that interval.

Survival analysis can also be done while controlling for confounding variables. The Cox Proportional Hazards model is a form of multivariate survival analysis which determines the "instantaneous mortality rate" at any given point in time, while controlling for other factors. Detailed exposition of Cox Proportional Hazards method is given in more technical and advanced texts.


## 5.7 Intention-to-Treat Analysis

Data from clinical trials in general should be analyzed by comparing the groups as they were originally randomized, and not by comparing to the placebo control group only those in the drug group who actually did take the drug. The people assigned to the active drug group should be included with that group for analysis even if they never took the drug. This may sound strange, since how can one assess the efficacy of a drug if the patient isn't taking it? But the very reason people may not comply to the drug regimen may have to do with adverse effects of the drug so that if we select out only those who do comply we have a different group from the one randomized and we may have a biased picture of the drug effects.

Another aspect is that there may be some quality of compliers in general, that affects outcome. A famous example of misleading conclusions which could arise from not doing an intention-to-treat analysis comes from the Coronary Drug Project[22]. This randomized, double-blind study compared the drug clofibrate to placebo for reducing cholesterol. The outcome variable, which was five-year mortality, was very similar in both groups, 18% in the drug group and 19% in the placebo group. It turned out however that only about two thirds of the patients who were supposed to take clofibrate, actually were compliant and did take their medication. These people had a 15% mortality rate, significantly lower than the 19% mortality in the placebo group. However, further analysis showed that among those assigned to the placebo group, one third didn't take their placebo pills either. The two thirds of the placebo group who were compliant had a mortality of 15%, just like the ones who complied to the clofibrate drug! The non-compliant people in both the drug and placebo groups had a higher mortality (25% for clofibrate and 28% for placebo). It may be desirable in some circumstances to look at the effect of a drug in those who actually take it. In that case the comparison of drug compliers should be to placebo compliers rather than to the placebo group as a whole.

The inclusion of non-compliers in the analysis dilutes the effects so every effort should be made to minimize non-compliance. In some trials a judged capacity for compliance is an enrollment criterion and an evaluation is made of every patient as part of determining his or her eligibility, as to whether this patient is likely to adhere to the regimen. Those not likely to do so are excluded prior to randomization. However, if the question at hand is how acceptable is the treatment to the patient, in addition to its efficacy, then the basis for inclusion may be the general population who might benefit from the drug, including the non-compliers.

## 5.8  How Large Should the Clinical Trial Be?

*A clinical trial should be large enough, i.e. have big enough sample size to have a high likelihood of detecting a true difference between the two groups.  If you do a small trial and find no significant difference, you have gained no new information;* you may not have found a difference simply because you didn't have enough people in the study.  You cannot make the statement that there is no difference between the treatments.  If you have a large trial and find no significant difference, then you are able to say with more certainty that the treatments are really not different.

Suppose you do find a significant difference in a small trial with $p < .05$ (level of significance).  This means that the result you obtained is likely to have arisen purely by chance less than 5 times in 100 (if there really were no difference). Is it to be trusted as much as the same p value from a large trial? There are several schools of thought about this.

The p value is an index of the strength of the evidence with regard to rejecting a null hypothesis. Some people think that a p value is a p value and carries the same weight regardless of whether it comes from a large or small study.  Others believe that if you get a significant result in a small trial, it means that the effect (or the difference between two population means) must be large enough so that you were able to detect it even with your small samples, and therefore, it is a meaningful difference.  It is true that if the sample size is large enough, we may find statistical significance if the real difference between means is very, very small and practically irrelevant.  Therefore, finding a significant difference in a small trial does mean that the effect was relatively large.

Still others say that in practice, however, you can have less confidence that the treatments really do differ for a given p value in a small trial than if you had obtained the same p value in testing these two treatments in a large trial.[24] This apparent paradox may arise in situations where there are many more small trials being carried out world-wide studying the same issue then there are large trials - such as in cancer therapy.  Some of those trials, by chance alone, will turn out to have significant results which may be misleading.

Suppose that there are 1000 small trials of anti-cancer drug therapy.  By chance alone, 5% of these will be significant even if the therapies have no effect, or 50 significant results.  Since these are by chance alone, it means we are incorrect to declare anti-cancer drug effects in these trials ( we have committed type I errors).  Suppose, further that there are only 100 large trials studying this same issue.  Of these, 5% or 5 such studies, will declare a difference to exist, incorrectly. So, if we combine all the trials which show significant differences *incorrectly*, we have 55 such significant but misleading, p values. Of these, 50 or 91% come from small trials and 5 out of the 55 incorrect ones (or 9%) come from the large trials. The following points are important:

1. There is a distinction between *statistical significance* and *clinical significance*. A result may not have arisen by chance, i.e. it may reflect a true difference, but be so small as to render it of no practical importance.

2. It is best to report the actual probability of obtaining the result by chance alone under the null hypothesis, i.e. the *actual p value*, rather than just saying it is significant or not. The p value for what we commonly call "significance" is arbitrary. By custom, it has been taken to be a p value of .05 or less. But the .05 cut point is not sacred. The reader should decide what strength he or she will put in the evidence provided by the study, and the reader must have the information to make that decision. The information must include: the design of the study, sample selection, the sample sizes, the standard deviations, and the actual p values.

*In summary*:

1. Finding *no significant difference* from a small trial tells us nothing.

2. Finding *no significant difference* in a large trial is a real finding and tells us the treatments are likely to be equivalent.

3. Finding a *significant difference* in a small trial may or may not be replicable.

4. Finding a *significant difference* in a large trial is to be trusted as revealing a true difference.

## 5.9  What Is Involved in Sample Size Calculation?

### a.  Effect size

Let us say that 15% of victims with a certain type of heart attack die if they are given drug A and 16% die if they are given drug B. Does this 1% difference mean drug A is better? Most people would say this is too small a difference, even if it doesn't arise by chance, to have any clinical importance. Suppose the difference between the two drugs is 5%. Would we now say drug A is better? That would depend on how large a difference we thought was important. *The size of the difference we want to detect is called the effect size.*

To calculate sample size you need to know the minimum size of the difference between two treatments that you would be willing to *miss* detecting. Suppose for example that in your control group 30% of the patients without the treatment recover. It is your belief that with treatment in the experimental group 40% will recover. You think this difference in recovery rate is clinically important and you want to be sure that you can detect a difference at least as large as the difference between 30% and 40%. This means that if the treatment group recovery rate were 35% you would be willing to miss finding that small an effect. However, if the treatment rate were 40% or more, you would want to be pretty sure to find it. How sure would you want to be? The issue of "how sure" has to do with the "power" of the statistical test.

## b.  Power

Statistical power means the *probability* of finding a real effect (of the size that you think is clinically important). The relationships among power, significance level and Type I and Type II error are summarized below:

  *Significance level = Probability of a Type I error* = Probability of finding an effect when there really isn't one. This is also known as alpha or $\alpha$.

  *Probability of Type II error* = probability of failing to find an effect when there really is one. This is also known as beta or $\beta$.

  *Power* = 1-Probability of Type II error = Probability of finding an effect when there really is one. This is also known as *1-beta*.

## c.  Sample size

*To calculate sample size, you have to specify your choice of effect size, significance level and desired power.* If you choose a significance level of .05 and a power of .80, then your Type II error probability is 1-power or .20. This means that you consider a Type I error to be 4 times more serious than a Type II error (.20/.05 = 4) or that you are 4 times as afraid of finding something that isn't there as of failing to find something that is. When you calculate sample size there is always a trade-off. If you want to decrease the probability of making a Type I error, then for a given sample size and effect size, you will increase the probability of making a Type II error. You can keep both types of error low by increasing your sample size. The table below shows the sample sizes necessary to compare two groups with a test between two proportions under different assumptions.

### SAMPLE SIZE EXAMPLES

| SIGNIFI-CANCE LEVEL (1-tail) | ASSUME: CONTROL GROUP RESPONSE RATE = | EFFECT SIZE DETECT INCREASE IN TREATMENT GROUP AT LEAST TO: | POWER WITH PROBA-BILITY OF: | SAMPLE SIZE N NEEDED IN EACH GROUP |
|---|---|---|---|---|
| .05 | 30% | 40% | .80 | 280 |
|     | 30% | 50% | .80 | 73 |
|     | 30% | 40% | .90 | 388 |
|     | 30% | 50% | .90 | 101 |
| .01 | 30% | 40% | .80 | 455 |
|     | 30% | 50% | .80 | 118 |
|     | 30% | 40% | .90 | 590 |
|     | 30% | 50% | .90 | 153 |

The second row of the table shows that if you want to be able to detect a difference in response rate from 30% in the control group to 50% or more in the treatment group with a probability (power) of .80, you would need 73 people in each of the two groups. If however, you want to be pretty sure that you find a difference as small as the one between 30% and 40%, then you must have 280 people in each group. If you want to be more sure of finding the difference, say 90% sure instead of 80% sure, then you will need 388 people in each group (rather than the 280 for .80 power). If you want to have a more stringent significance level of .01, you will need 118 people in each group (compared to the 73 needed for the .05 significance level) to be able to detect the difference between 30% and 50%; you will need 455 people (compared to 280 for the .05 level) to detect a difference from 30% to 40% response rate.

The table below shows the impact on sample size of a one-tail test of significance versus a two-tail test. Recall that a two-tail test postulates that the response rate in the treatment group can be *either larger or smaller* than the response rate in the control group, while a one-tail test specifies the direction of the hypothesized difference. *A two-tail test requires a larger sample size*, but that is the one most commonly used.

### SAMPLE SIZE EXAMPLES

| SIGNIFI-CANCE LEVEL = .05 | ASSUME: CONTROL GROUP RESPONSE RATE = | EFFECT SIZE DETECT INCREASE IN TREATMENT GROUP AT LEAST TO: | POWER WITH PROBA-BILITY OF: | SAMPLE SIZE n NEEDED IN EACH GROUP |
|---|---|---|---|---|
| 1-TAIL | 30% | 40% | .80 | 280 |
| 2-TAIL | 30% | 40% | .80 | 356 |
| 1-TAIL | 30% | 50% | .80 | 73 |
| 2-TAIL | 30% | 50% | .80 | 92 |

### d. Some additional considerations

For a fixed sample size and a given effect size, or difference you want to detect, maximum power occurs when the event rate is about 50%. So to maximize power it may sometimes be wise to select a group for study which is likely to have the events of interest. For example, if you want to study the effects of a beta-blocker drug on preventing heart attacks, you could get "more power for the money" by studying persons who have already had one heart attack rather than healthy persons, since the former are more likely to have another event (heart attack). Of course you might then be looking at a different question: the effect of beta-blockers on survivors of heart attack, rather than the effect of beta-blockers in preventing the first heart attack. Clearly judgment is required.

### 5.10 How to Calculate Sample Size for the Difference Between Two Proportions

You need to specify what you think the proportion of events is likely to be in each of the two groups being compared. An event may be a response, a death, a recovery - but it must be a dichotomous variable. Your specification of the event rates in the two groups reflects the size of the difference you would like to be able to detect.

Specify:

$p_1$ = rate in group 1;    $q_1 = 1 - p_1$;    alpha = significance level

$p_2$ = rate in group 2;    $q_2 = 1 - p_2$;    power

$$n = \frac{(p_1 q_1) + (p_2 q_2)}{(p_2 - p_1)^2} \times f(alpha, power)$$

The values of f (alpha, power) for a two-tail test can be obtained from the table below.

VALUES OF f (alpha, power)

|  |  | .95 | .90 | .80 | .50 |
|---|---|---|---|---|---|
| alpha significance level .01 | .10 | 10.8 | 8.6 | 6.2 | 2.7 |
| | .05 | 13.0 | 10.5 | 7.9 | 3.8 |
| | .01 | 17.8 | 14.9 | 11.7 | 6.6 |

NOTE:  n is roughly inversely proportional to $(p_2 - p_1)^2$

Example:

Suppose you want to find the sample size to detect a difference from 30% to 40% between 2 groups, with a power of .80 and a significance level of .05. Then,

$p_1 = .30 \quad q_1 = .70 \quad$ alpha = .05
$p_2 = .40 \quad q_2 = .60 \quad$ power = .80

f(alpha, power) = 7.9 from the table

$$n = \frac{(.30)(.70) + (.40)(.60)}{(.40 - .30)^2} \times 7.9 = 356$$

You would need 356 people in each group to be 80% sure you can detect a difference from 30% to 40% at the .05 level.

## 5.11  How to Calculate Sample Size for Testing the Difference Between Two Means

The formula to calculate sample size for a test of the difference between two means, assuming there is to be an equal number in each group, is:

$$n = \frac{k \times 2\sigma^2}{(MD)^2} = \textit{number in each group}$$

$\sigma^2$ is the error variance.
MD is the minimum difference one wishes to detect.
k depends on the significance level and power desired.

Selected values of k are shown below.

| Significance Level | Power | k |
|---|---|---|
| .05 | .99 | 18.372 |
| | .95 | 12.995 |
| | .90 | 10.507 |
| | .80 | 7.849 |
| .01 | .99 | 24.031 |
| | .95 | 17.814 |
| | .90 | 14.879 |
| | .80 | 11.679 |

For example to detect a difference in mean I.Q. of 5 points between two groups of people, where the variance $= 16^2 = 256$, at a significance level of .05 and with power of .80, we would need

$$n = \frac{7.849 \times 2(256)}{(5)^2} = 161 \textit{ people}$$

in each group or a total sample size of 322. This means we are 80% likely to detect a difference as large or larger than 5 points. For a 10 point difference, we would need 54 people in each group.

A common set of parameters for such sample size calculations are $\alpha = .05$ and power $= .80$. However, when there are multiple comparisons, we have to set $\alpha$ at lower levels as described in Section 3.22 on the Bonferroni procedure. Then our sample size would need to be greater.

If we are hoping to show that two treatments are equivalent, we have to set the minimum difference we want to detect to be very small and the power to be very, very high, resulting in very large sample sizes.

To calculate values of k which are not tabulated here, the reader is referred to the book *Methods in Observational Epidemiology* by Kelsey, Thompson and Evans for an excellent explanation.

## 5.12  The Impact of Epidemiology on Human Lives

Ten years ago a woman with breast cancer would be likely to have a radical mastectomy, which in addition to removal of the breast and the resulting disfigurement, would also include removal of much of the muscle wall in her chest and leave her incapacitated in many ways. Today, hardly anyone gets a radical mastectomy and many don't even get a modified mastectomy, but, depending on the cancer, may get a lumpectomy which just removes the lump, leaving the breast intact. Years ago, no one paid much attention to radon, an inert gas released from the soil and dissipated through foundation cracks into homes - now it is recognized as a leading cause of lung cancer. The role of nutrition in prevention of disease was not recognized by the scientific community. In fact, people who believed in the importance of nutrients in the cause and cure of disease were thought to be faddists, just a bit nutty. Now it is frequently the subject of articles, books and news items, and substantial sums of research monies are invested in nutritional studies.

In the health field changes in treatment, prevention and prevailing knowledge come about when there is a confluence of circumstances: new information is acquired to supplant existing theories; there is dissemination of this information to the scientific community and to the public at large; and, there is the appropriate psychological, economic and political climate which would welcome the adoption of the new approaches. Epidemiology plays a major role by providing the methods by which new scientific knowledge is acquired. Often, the first clues to causality come long before a biological mechanism is known. Around 1850 in London, Dr. John Snow, dismayed at the suffering an deaths caused by epidemics of cholera, carefully studied reports of such epidemics and noted that cholera was much more likely to occur in certain parts of London than in other parts. He mapped the places where cholera was rampant and where it was less so, and he noted that houses supplied with water by one company, the Southwark and Vauxhall Company, had many more cases of cholera than those supplied by another company. He also knew that the Vauxhall Company used as its source an area heavily contaminated by sewage. Snow insisted that the city close the pump supplying the contaminated water - known as the Broad Street Pump. They did so and cholera abated. All this was 25 years before anyone isolated the cholera bacillus and long before people accepted the notion that disease could be spread by water. In modern times, the AIDS epidemic is one where the method of spread was identified before the infectious agent, the HIV virus was known.

Epidemiological techniques have been increasingly applied to chronic diseases, which differ from infectious diseases in that they may persist for a long time (while infections usually either kill quickly or are cured quickly) and also usually have multiple causes many of which are difficult to identify. Here, also epidemiology plays a central role in identifying risk factors such as smoking for lung cancer for instance. Such knowledge is translated into public action before the full biological pathways are elucidated. The action takes the form of educational campaigns, anti-smoking laws, restrictions on advertisement and other mechanisms to limit smoking. The risk factors for heart disease have been identified through classic epidemiologic studies resulting in lifestyle changes for individuals as well as public policy consequences.

Chronic diseases present different and challenging problems in analysis and new statistical techniques continue to be developed to accommodate such problems. Thus the field of statistic is not static and the field of epidemiology is not fixed. Both adapt and expand to deal with the changing health problems of our society.

# BIBLIOGRAPHY

1. Popper KR: The Logic of Scientific Discovery. New York: Harper and Row, 1959.

2. Weed DL: On the Logic of Causal Inference, American Journal of Epidemiology 123(6):965-979, 1985.

3. Goodman SN, Royall R: Evidence and Scientific Research, AJPH, 78(12):1568-1574, 1988.

4. Susser M: Rules of Inference in Epidemiology. <u>Regulatory Toxicology and Pharmacology</u>, Academic Press, Inc., Chapter 6, pp. 116-128, 1986.

5. Brown HI: Perception, Theory and Commitment: The New Philosophy of Science, Chicago, Precedent, 1977.

6. Principles of Medical Statistics, Sir Bradford Hill, Oxford University Press, 9th Edition, NY, 1971.

7. Health, United States, 1987, Pub. No. (PHS) 88-1232, Public Health Service, Hyattsville, MD, 1988.

8. Drapkin A, Mersky C: Anticoagulant Therapy after Acute Myocardial Infarction. JAMA, 222:541-548, 1972.

9. Intellectual Development of Children: U.S. Department of Health, Education, and Welfare, Public Health Service, HSMHA, December 1971, Vital and Health Statistics Series 11 - November 10.

10. Davis BR, Blaufox MD, Hawkins CM, Langford HG, Oberman A, Swencionis C, Wassertheil-Smoller S, Wylie-Rosett J, Zimbaldi N: Trial of Antihypertensive Interventions and Management. Design, Methods, and Selected Baseline Results. Cont. Clin. Trials, 10:11-30, 1989.

11. Oberman A, Wassertheil-Smoller S, Langford H, Blaufox MD, Davis BR, Blaszkowski T, Zimbaldi N, Hawkins CM, for the TAIM Group: Pharmacologic and Nutritional Treatment of Mild Hypertension: Changes in Cardiovascular Risk Status. Annals of Internal Medicine, January, 1990.

12. Rothman KJ: No Adjustments are Needed for Multiple Comparisons. Epidemiology 1(1):43-46, 1990.

13.Scarr-Salapateck S: Race, Social Class, and I.Q.. Science, 174:1285-1295, 1971.

14.Sokal RR, Rohlf JF: Biometry. W.H. Freeman and Co., San Francisco, 1969.

15.NCHS: Advanced Report of Final Mortality Statistics, 1987, Supl. (p. 12), MSVR Vol. 38, No. 5, Pub. No. (PHS) 89-1120, Public Health Service, Hyattsville, MD, September 26, 1989.

16.Hypertension Detection and Follow-Up Program Cooperative Group: Blood Pressure Studies in 14 Communities. A Two-Stage Screen for Hypertension. JAMA, 237(22):2385-2391, 1977.

17.Inter-Society Commission for Heart Disease Resources. Atherosclerosis Study Group and Epidemiology Study Group: Primary Prevention of the Atherosclerotic Diseases. Circulation, 42:A55, 1970.

18.Meyer KB, Pauker SG: Screening for HIV: Can We Afford the False Postive Rate? NEJM 317(4):238-241, 1987.

19.The Framingham Study: An Epidemiological Investigation of Cardiovascular Disease. W.B. Kannel and T. Gordon (eds). Feb. 1974, DHEW Publ. No. (NIH) 74-599.

20.These data come from the National Pooling Project. For purposes of this example, high blood pressure is defined as diastolic blood pressure $\geq 105$Hg and "normal" is defined as DPB$< 78$ mmHg. The disease in question is a "Coronary Event" and the time periods is 10 years.

21.Lilienfeld AM: Foundations of Epidemiological, Oxford University Press, 1976, p. 180.

22.Coronary Drug Project Research Group: Influence of Adherence to Treatment and Response of Cholesterol on Mortality in the Coronary Drug Project. NEJM 303:1038-1041, 1980.

23.The numerical example is due to the courtesy of Dr. Martin Lesser, Cornell University Medical Center.

24.Peto R, Pike MC, Armitage P, Breslow NE, Cox DR, Howard SV, Mantel N, McPherson K, Peto J, Smith PG: Design and Analysis of Randomized Clinical Trials Requiring Prolonged Observation of Each Patient. I. Introduction and Design. Br. J. Cancer, 34:585-612, 1976.

# APPENDIX A

Critical Values of Chi-Square, z, and t.

When z, $\chi^2$ or t value calculated from the observed data is equal to or exceeds THE CRITICAL VALUE listed below, we can reject the null hypothesis at the given significance level, $\alpha$ (alpha).

## Selected Critical Values of Chi-Square

| Significance Level | .1 | .05 | .01 | .001 |
|---|---|---|---|---|
| Critical Value of $\chi^2$ | 2.71 | 3.84 | 6.63 | 10.83 |

## Selected Critical Values of Z

| Significance Level Two-Tail Test (One-Tail Test | .1 (.05) | .05 (.025) | .01 (.005) | .001 (.0005) |
|---|---|---|---|---|
| Critical Value of Z | 1.64 | 1.96 | 2.58 | 3.29 |

## Selected Critical Values of t

| Significance Level Two-Tail Test (One-Tail) | .10 (.05) | .05 (.025) | .01 (.005) | .001 (.0005) |
|---|---|---|---|---|
| Degrees of Freedom | | | | |
| 9 | 1.83 | 2.26 | 3.25 | 4.78 |
| 19 | 1.73 | 2.09 | 3.86 | 3.88 |
| 100 | 1.66 | 1.98 | 2.63 | 3.39 |
| 1000 | 1.64 | 1.96 | 2.58 | 3.29 |

NOTE: Interpretation:
If you have 19 degrees of freedom, to reject $H_o$, at $\alpha$ = .05 with a two-tailed test you would need a value of t as large or larger than 2.09; for $\alpha$ = .01, a t at least as large as 3.86 would be needed. Note that when df gets very large the critical values of t are the same as the critical values of Z. Values other than those calculated here appear in most of the texts shown in the book list.

# APPENDIX B

## How to Calculate A Correlation Coefficient

| Individual | XY | X | Y | $X^2$ | $Y^2$ |
|---|---|---|---|---|---|
| A | 5 | 7 | 25 | 49 | 35 |
| B | 8 | 4 | 64 | 16 | 32 |
| C | 15 | 8 | 225 | 64 | 120 |
| D | 20 | 10 | 400 | 100 | 200 |
| E | 25 | 14 | 625 | 196 | 350 |
| | 73 | 43 | 1339 | 425 | 737 |

$$r = \frac{N\Sigma XY - (\Sigma X)(\Sigma Y)}{\sqrt{N\Sigma X^2 - (\Sigma X)^2}\ \sqrt{N\Sigma Y^2 - (\Sigma Y)^2}}$$

$$= \frac{5(737) - (73)(43)}{\sqrt{5(1339) - (73)^2}\ \sqrt{5(425) - (43)^2}} = \frac{3685 - 3139}{\sqrt{1366}\ \sqrt{276}}$$

$$= \frac{546}{(37)(16.6)} = \frac{546}{614} = .89$$

# APPENDIX C

**How to calculate regression coefficients.**

| Individual | X | Y | $X^2$ | $Y^2$ | XY |
|---|---|---|---|---|---|
| A | 5 | 7 | 25 | 49 | 35 |
| B | 8 | 4 | 64 | 16 | 32 |
| C | 15 | 8 | 225 | 64 | 120 |
| D | 20 | 10 | 400 | 100 | 200 |
| E | 25 | 14 | 625 | 196 | 350 |
|   | 73 | 43 | 1339 | 425 | 737 |

$$b = \frac{\Sigma XY - \dfrac{(\Sigma X)(\Sigma Y)}{N}}{\Sigma X^2 - \dfrac{(\Sigma X)^2}{N}}$$

$$a = \Sigma \frac{Y}{N} - b \frac{\Sigma X}{N}$$

$$b = \frac{737 - \dfrac{(73)(43)}{5}}{1339 - \dfrac{(73)^2}{5}} = \frac{737 - 628}{1339 - 1066} = \frac{109}{273} = .40$$

$$a = \frac{43}{5} - \frac{.40(73)}{5} = 8.60 - 5.84 = 2.76$$

# APPENDIX D

**Age-Adjustment**

Consider two populations: A and B with the following characteristics:

| Popula-tion | Age | Age Specific Rates | Number of People in Population | Number of Deaths in Population | Crude Death Rate |
|---|---|---|---|---|---|
| A | Young | $\frac{4}{1000}$ = .004 | 500 | .004 x 500 = 2 | |
| | Old | $\frac{16}{1000}$ = .016 | 500 | .016 x 500 = 8 | |
| | Total | | 1000 | 10 | $\frac{10}{1000}$ |
| B | Young | $\frac{5}{1000}$ = .005 | 667 | .005 x 667 = 3.335 | |
| | Old | $\frac{20}{1000}$ = .020 | 333 | .020 x 333 = 6.665 | |
| | Total | | 1000 | 10 | $\frac{10}{1000}$ |

Note that the population B has higher age-specific death rates in each age group than population A, but both populations have the same crude death rate of 10/1000. The reason for this is that population A has a greater proportion of old people (50%) and even though the death rate for the old people is 16/1000 in population A compared to 20/1000 in population B, the greater number of people in that group contribute to a greater number of total deaths.

To perform age adjustment, we must select a standard population to which we will compare both A and B. The following examples use two different standard populations as illustrations. In practice, a standard population is chosen either as the population during a particular year or as the combined A and B population. The choice of standard population does not matter. The phrase "standard population" in this context refers to a population with a particular age distribution (if we are adjusting for age) or sex distribution (if we are adjusting for sex). The age-specific (or sex-specific, if that is what is being adjusted) rates for both group A and B are applied to the age distribution of the standard population in order to compare A and B *as if* they had the same age distribution.

## STANDARD POPULATION I

Example: (More old people
than young)

| Age | Number of People | | Apply age specific death rates for *Population A* to standard population | | No of deaths expected in A *if it were the same age composition* as the standard population | Apply age specific death rates for *Population B* to standard population | No of deaths expected in B *if it were the same age composition* as the standard population |
|------|------|---|------|---|------|------|------|
| Young | 300 | x | .004 | = | 1.2 | .005 | 1.5 |
| Old | 700 | x | .016 | = | 11.2 | .020 | 14. |
| Total | 1000 | | | | 12.4 | | 15.5 |

| Age-adjusted rates for: A = 12/1000 | B = 15/1000 |

## STANDARD POPULATION II

Example:  (More young people
than old)

| Age | Number of People | | Apply age specific rates for *A* to standard population | | No of deaths expected in A if it were the same age composition as the standard population | Apply age specific rates for *B* to standard population | No of deaths expected in B |
|------|------|---|------|---|------|------|------|
| Young | 1167 | x | .004 | = | 4.67 | .005 | 5.84 |
| Old | 833 | x | .016 | = | 13.33 | .020 | 16.66 |
| Total | 2000 | | | | 18 | | 22.50 |

Age-adjusted rates for: A = $\dfrac{18}{2000}$

$= \dfrac{9}{1000}$

B = $\dfrac{22.50}{2000} = \dfrac{11.25}{1000}$

Note if you use 2 different standard populations you get different age-adjusted rates *but* relative figures are same, i.e. the age-adjusted rates for A are lower than for B. This implies that the age-specific rates for A are lower than for B, but since the crude rates are the same, it must mean that population A is older. Because we know that age specific rates for older people are higher than for younger people, population A must have been weighted by a larger proportion of older people (who contributed more deaths) in order to result in the same crude rate as B but in a lower age adjusted rate.

There are exceptions to the above inference when we consider groups where infant mortality is very high. In that case it could be that the young have very high death rates, even higher than the old. In industrialized societies, however, the age-specific death rates for the old are higher than for the young.

# APPENDIX E
## Confidence Limits on Odds Ratios

The 95% confidence limits for an odds ratio (OR) are:

$$O.R. \times e^{\left[\pm 1.96\sqrt{\frac{1}{a} + \frac{1}{b} + \frac{1}{c} + \frac{1}{d}}\right]}$$

We reproduce here the table from Section 4.13 to use as an example:

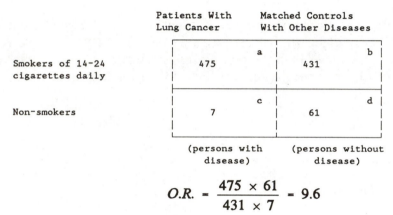

|  | Patients With Lung Cancer | Matched Controls With Other Diseases |
|---|---|---|
| Smokers of 14-24 cigarettes daily | a 475 | b 431 |
| Non-smokers | c 7 | d 61 |
|  | (persons with disease) | (persons without disease) |

$$O.R. = \frac{475 \times 61}{431 \times 7} = 9.6$$

Upper 95% confidence limit =

$$O.R. \times e^{\left[1.96\sqrt{\frac{1}{475} + \frac{1}{431} + \frac{1}{7} + \frac{1}{6}}\right]}$$

$$O.R. \times e^{[1.96(.128)]} = 9.6 \times e^{(.25)} = 9.6 \times 1.28 = 12.3$$

Lower 95% confidence limit =

$$O.R. \times e^{[-1.96(.128)]} = 9.6 \times e^{-.25} = 9.6 \times .78 = 7.5$$

$$NOTE: \quad e^{-.25} = \frac{1}{e^{-.25}} = .78$$

Thus the confidence interval is 7.5 to 12.3

# BOOK TITLES

1. Anderson S, Auquier A, Hauck WW, Oakes D, Vandaele W, Weisberg HI: Statistical Methods for Comparative Studies. Don Wylie and Sons, NY 1980.

   Intermediate Level. Requires a prior course in statistics. Excellent for applied researchers.

2. Bradford Hill, Sir Austin, Statistical Methods in Clinical and Preventive Medicine, E.S. Livingstone Ltd., Edinburgh and London, 1962.

   Classic text on the subject.

3. Campbell, DT and Cook, TD: Quasiexperimentation: Design and Analysis for Field Settings, Rand McNally, Chicago, 1979.

   This book focuses on the design and measurement issues, particularly types of bias, which can arise in quasi-experimental studies. It also deals with the appropriate statistical techniques to be used. The book is particularly relevant to persons interested in program evaluation.

4. Cohen J: Statistical Power Analysis for the Behavioral Sciences. Second Edition. Lawrence Erlbaum Assoc. Publishers, Hillsdale, NJ 1988.

   A classic and a must. Everything you ever wanted to know about sample size calculations, clearly and comprehensively explained. A reference and source book. Probably needs to be interpreted by a statistician.

5. Colton, T: Statistics in Medicine, Little Brown and Company, Boston, 1974.

   A good first level statistics text.

6. Elwood JM: Causal Relationships in Medicine. A Practical System for Critical Appraisal. Oxford University Press, NY, 1988.

   Excellent book with clear explanations of study designs, epidemiological concepts and relevant statistical methods.

7.      Fleiss, JL:  Statistical Methods for Rates and Proportions, Second
        Edition, John Wiley and Sons, New York, 1982.

        An excellent second level statistics text concerned with the analysis of
        qualitative or categorical data.


8.      Fleiss, JL:  The Design and Analysis of Clinical Experiments, John Wiley
        and Sons, New York, 1986.

        The book focuses on the technical aspects of the design and statistical
        analysis of experimental studies.

9.      Fryer HPC:  Concepts and Methods of Experimental Statistics.  Allyn &
        Bacon Inc., Boston, 1966.

        Basic detailed book on statistical methods.  Intermediate to higher
        level.  Many formulae and symbols.  More in-depth statistics.

10.     Hosmer DW, Lemeshow S:  Applied Logistic Regression.  John Wylie &
        Sons, NY, 1989.

        Advanced book on model building in logistic regression, requires
        statistical background.

11.     Ingelfinger JA, Mosteller F, Thibodeau LA, Ware JH:  Biostatistics in
        Clinical Medicine.  Maxmillen Publishing Co., NY, 1983.

        Mostly aimed at physicians.  Intermediate level.  Very good
        explanations of biostatistics.  Many examples from research
        literature.

12.     Kahn HA:  An Introduction to Epidemiologic Methods.  Oxford
        University Press, NY, 1983.

        Intermediate level book on epidemiologic and selected statistical
        methods.  Good explanations of life table analysis and multiple
        regression and multiple logistic functions.  Clear explanations of
        longitudinal studies using person years.

13.     Kelsey JL, Thompson WD, Evans AS:  Methods in Observational Epidemiology.  Oxford University Press, 1986.

        Extremely useful explanations of issues involved in case-control, retrospective and prospective studies.  A good discussion of matching, stratification, and design issues.

14.     Kleinbaum DG, Kupper LL, Morgenstern E:  Epidemiologic Research Principles and Quantitative Methods.  Wasdworth, Belmont, CA, 1982.

        An advanced text designed primarily for persons conducting observational epidemiologic research.  Both design and statistical issues are covered.

15.     Kleinbaum DG, Kupper LL:  Applied Regression Analysis and Other Multi-variable Methods.  Wadsworth, Belmont, CA, 1978.

        This text, as the title indicates, deals with multiple regression and allied topics.

16.     Popcock SJ:  Clinical Trials:  A Practical Approach, John Wiley and Sons, New York, 1983

        An excellent book for anyone undertaking a clinical trial.

17.     Riegelman RK:  Studying a Study and Testing a Test:  How to Read the Medical Literature, Little Brown and Company, Boston, 1981.

        An introduction to epidemiologic methods and principles aimed at clinicians.

18.     Rothman KJ:  Modern Epidemiology, Little Brown and Company, Boston, 1986.

        An advanced text which covers both design and statistical issues.  The focus is an observational epidemiological study and is directed at the researcher more than the clinician.

19.     Sackett DL, Haynes RB, Tugwell P:  Clinical Epidemiology:  A Basic Science for Clinical Medicine.  Little Brown and Company, Boston, 1985.

The focus in this book is on applications of epidemiology in clinical practice.

20. Siegel, S: Nonparametric Statistics for the Behavioral Sciences, McGraw-Hill, NY, Toronto, London, 1956.

A "how-to-do-it" book; an excellent reference; outlines each procedure step-by-step, a classic.

21. Sokal RR, Rohlf JF: Biometry, W.H. Freeman and Company, San Francisco, 1969.

Rather complex and comprehensive.

# INDEX

Date Due